# Purpose High

## *Living with Autism*

An Up-Close and Candid Conversation
About Autism and Faith

# Mirian T. Sansalone

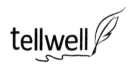

Tellwell Talent
www.tellwell.ca

ISBN
978-1-77302-583-4 (Paperback)
978-1-77302-582-7 (eBook)

# Table of Contents

# DEDICATION

Heavenly Father, I dedicate this book to you.

It was written for you, as a love letter. The story has been scripted in reverence to you; every word has the purpose of glorifying your name. I am humbled and grateful that you have placed these thoughts in my mind and in my heart.

I love you Father. This is for you.

# ACKNOWLEDGEMENTS

Gian, when we got married, I thought I could not love you more than I loved you then. But after month after year after birth after graduation of our four beautiful children, I knew I was wrong. Today, my love for you is deeper, my respect higher. So if I can wake up every morning to the harsh reality of non-verbal autism and if I can go to bed to the inherent and all-consuming pain of disability and see God smiling back at me, it is because of you. You are the reason why I can laugh and I can love and I can hope. There are twenty chapters and an epilogue in this book. This number is on purpose, for you. Your kidney transplant surgery dates back to August 20, 1980. Twenty, plus one for good luck. I do not know how to love you more, Gian, but if there is a way, I will find it, and then, I will love you more.

Domenico, Roberto, Rocco, and Jennifer, you make my heart grow wings. You are light and life, love and virtue. You are everything.

Rocco and Jennifer, I put you before your brothers this time. Every other time in your lives, I have put them first. And I don't know where to start, because there is no end. There will never be enough space to say everything I want to say to you. Living with autism is all you have ever known. I hope and pray that my actions speak to the gratitude and respect I have for you. Roc and Jen, my hands, they work for you. My smile, it calls out your name. My heart is full because you live there; you are my home.

Domenico and Roberto, in the pages and chapters of this book, I celebrate you. In my daily labour, I honour you. My final word and my last breath will be in advocacy for you. I will neither rest nor sleep until I see you reach that sacred place God has prepared for you. We will solve the autism puzzle together, one piece at a time.

Laura, you laboured with me through ten edits of *Purpose High*, heart to heart. You made the time to dream with me and you never gave up on me. You helped me organize my thoughts. You gave me confidence, turning "I think" into "I know". I came to believe in myself because you believed in me. My life is good because of you, Laura. You are forever LG.

Paula, you bring grace to your noble and chosen profession. You work for the people, and uphold the right to be truly human, visible, and connected. You taught me about the power of positivity. It is the greatest life skill and you live it, every single day. It was from you I learned that there are many different ways to do the same thing. You have been a mentor and a friend and for that, there are no words.

Anthony, thank you for the gentle manner in which you put the brakes on *Purpose High*, so it could fly higher. You gave generously of your talents and your time. How does one say thank you for that?

To you, the reader - friends I know and friends I hope to meet - thank you for spending this time with me. I am honoured and excited. I want to make you laugh and reflect and believe that you too have a story. Tell it to yourself; tell it to the world. Live it, own it, and do it with purpose!

# Chapter One

## LIFE BEFORE PLAN B

*Sometimes on the way to your dream,*
*you get lost and find a better one.*

**LISA HAMMOND**

Give me a minute. This is tough. Nothing comes to mind. I cannot remember life before Plan B, life before autism.

Plan A - get an education, get married, have a family, raise my children, excel in my career, live happily ever after. Something like that, right? Try again, Mirian. Living with autism is all about Plan B.

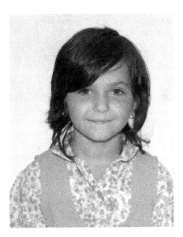

Mini me, 1972

Born and raised in Canada, I am fifty-three years old. I spoke both English and Italian until I started Junior Kindergarten. Once in school, English became my first language. I live in a small town in Southern Ontario with my husband and our four children. Domenico, Roberto, Rocco, and Jennifer remain my life's greatest labour of love.

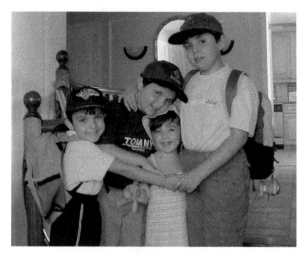

My life's greatest labour of love

My husband Giancarlo of twenty-eight years strong is my partner in life and love and, by a wide margin, my most trusted friend.

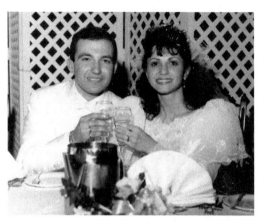

And they lived happily ever after, October 29, 1988

Domenico and Roberto are my eldest children, aged twenty-five and twenty-two respectively. Both have autism. Rocco and Jennifer are twenty and nineteen, developing normally, and sending me directly to the funny farm. Do not pass go, do not collect two hundred dollars.

So how do I make it work and how do I make it count? How do I bring together the pervasive world of autism and the conventional reality of the typical family unit in perfect sync? How do I maintain a sense of autonomy, a sense of self in the midst of perpetual chaos?

Before going any further, can we talk?

As an adolescent, I struggled with clutter in my head. It littered my thoughts. I was confused and had no direction in life. After a failed attempt at post-secondary education, I eventually developed some employable skills, found a job, and got married. I was finally grounded and focused on the future. I was excited to start a family. After eighteen cycles of infertility treatments followed by a laparoscopy, I experienced success! We were expecting our first child, finally. I was so happy. We were so happy. Only eight treatments for baby number two. Baby number three came after six treatments. Domenico, Roberto, and Rocco were all conceived with the aid of modern medicine. How romantic!

At that point in my life, family planning was the last thing on my mind. Since the age of seventeen, my menstrual cycle had been irregular, sometimes absent. Conception was only possible through medical intervention. Following the births of my three sons, a normal menstrual cycle did not resume. No chance of an unplanned pregnancy, I reassured myself. When Rocco was six months old, my menstrual cycle came unexpectedly out of hibernation. *You have been asleep for so long, and now you decide to inconvenience me? Gee, thanks. Thanks a lot.* Six weeks later, I felt nauseated. Baby number four, our daughter Jennifer, was born in November. She was God's idea. What other intentions did God have for my life?

I always wanted to have a strong relationship with God. My entire educational experience had been with the public school board, and I felt I had missed out on my spiritual development. When I was old enough to drive myself, I attended Sunday mass regularly. I was eager to learn about God. I wanted to be a practicing parishioner. I wanted to listen to the word of God and live by His instruction. But I stopped going to mass the day Plan B was imposed.

Autism was God's way of harnessing my complete and undivided attention. I know that now. I did not know that when I received Domenico's diagnosis. But perhaps it is not for the human mind or heart to understand everything that happens in this life. Maybe God guides us into His Light in His time and in His way. Maybe a life with God means that some of our questions will remain unanswered. Living with autism has raised so many questions over the years. There is one question, however, that resonates above the silence of non-verbal autism. This question speaks volumes. If you are curious, keep reading.

Lesson learned - Life always gives you a way out, a second chance: Plan B!

# Chapter Two

## MY WILL BE DONE

*We were born to make manifest the glory of God that is within us.*

MARIANNE WILLIAMSON

What gives life purpose? For me, the answer is a life of service. I wanted to be a nurse. I was enrolled in the baccalaureate degree program at the University of Toronto, Faculty of Nursing. I had accepted the scholarship. I was living the dream, my dream, when an overwhelming feeling of panic and self-doubt quickly took hold of me. Just two months into the program, I quit. I became a part-time student, successfully completing the two elective courses that I was already registered in as a requirement of the program. I reapplied for the next academic year, was reaccepted, and quit a second time. I then applied to the diploma nursing program at George Brown College in Toronto, was accepted, and quit in the first month. To stop the humiliating cycle of student one day, drop-out the next, I walked away from that dream. I felt like a failure. I sought employment as a medical secretary following some rudimentary training.

I first worked in a dental office as a Medical Dictaphone Transcriptionist. The orthodontist would belt out his treatment reports into a tape recorder. I would listen to the dictation and type it out in letter format for the next day. That was one of the perks of the job. I never had to see my boss; I just had to listen to him talk. And I could turn him off at any time. He always started his letters to colleagues in the same way: "Dear Dr. Toothless, I had the pleasure of meeting Master Gummy Smile or Madam Mixed Dentition today. Thank you for your kind referral." Under my breath and sometimes out loud, I thanked my boss for boring me to death, again. My office was in the basement. Who would hear me? But it was a job within the health care profession, and so I convinced myself it was a good start. I later accepted a position at a hospital in the Nursing Administration Department. *That was more like it!* After getting married, I found a job closer to our new home in Staff Development, not the department of my choice, but I was working in a hospital. *Good enough for now.* I was learning new skills, networking with colleagues, becoming integrated in the hospital setting, and building a life. Plan A was unfolding. Not exactly as anticipated, but I was moving in a forward direction. Then Plan B came along. Autism. Plan B dominated.

I was in the second trimester of my third pregnancy when a diagnosis of autism was delivered. It was just Domenico, Rocco in uterus, and me, waiting in the doctor's office to receive the news that Domenico has autism. I was still working at the time. I abandoned Plan A immediately. I quit my job. I took all of my vacation time, a leave of absence, an early maternity leave, and never looked back. I inherently understood that I had a different job to do. I had been given more than I could have ever imagined. I had not signed on for this think-outside-the-box kind of living.

I have no title, no letters after my name to speak of, no skill set, and no area of expertise. Instead, I have the awesome responsibility of making life-changing decisions for my sons, Domenico and Roberto.

If given the opportunity, would I go back to that university lecture hall; would I stay the course? If I could sit across the table from God and be granted "My will be done" rather than "Thy will be done" as declared in The Lord's Prayer, would I know how to respond? Good question; thanks for asking. Stay tuned: I will get to that later.

Many members of my inner circle have encouraged me to share my life's labour. At first, I quickly dismissed the thought of writing a book about living with autism. *Family and friends were just being kind*, I told myself. The unrelenting voice inside my head insisted *you don't have the know-how, Mirian.* But then virtual strangers reiterated the same sentiment. Year after year the message seemed unanimous, "You should write a book." How could so many people be wrong? I was finally persuaded. It was a good idea.

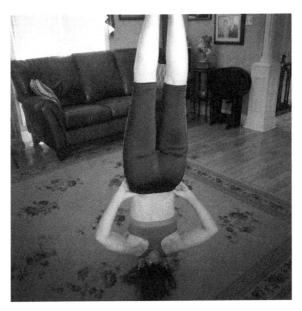

Just when I thought I had life all figured out

I am just an ordinary person. My story is not a tale of miracles. It is a story of finding purpose in your pain, facing your fears, and always seeing the glass half full. My personal journey of faith has taken me from obstacle to triumph, setback to milestone, confusion to realization, and back again, where at every corner and at each stop I have found myself looking at the many different faces of autism and seeing God smiling back at me.

Lesson learned - The only mistakes we make are the ones we learn nothing from. All other mistakes are lessons. Lessons are the building blocks to a fulfilling life.

# Chapter Three

## THE DIAGNOSTIC PROCESS

---

*There are some people who could hear you speak a*
*thousand words and still not understand you.*
*And there are others who will understand*
*without you even speaking a word.*

---

**UNKNOWN**

No parent should have to beg for a diagnosis. I had to. I had to *beg*. I
knew something was wrong.

I did not know that atypical play skills were suggestive of an Autism
Spectrum Disorder (ASD). I did not make the connection between
a lack of eye contact and delays in both social and language development. My observations of repetitive behaviour did not raise any red
flags. I was trying to enjoy the child I never thought I would have
because of infertility issues. But when Domenico was not talking in
sentences at an age when he should have been, I knew he needed help.
By the time of his third birthday, I became very concerned about his
language and communication skills. Four visits to Domenico's paediatrician finally fueled the process of obtaining a diagnosis.

I had first visited our paediatrician to request a referral to a speech and language pathologist. Domenico had a vocabulary of twenty words by the time he was two-and-a-half years old. Our paediatrician assured me that, in general, male children develop later than female children. I left his office without the referral.

I returned a second time, several months later. I wanted to have Domenico's hearing tested, since he would not respond to his name when he was called. Our paediatrician dismissed my concerns as nonsensical. He suggested that Domenico was withdrawing after the birth of our second son, Roberto. Domenico would come around. I left his office without the referral, again.

My third visit's objective was in response to Domenico's gross motor delays and behaviour. He was still not walking. He was not demonstrating appropriate play behaviour for his age. He always chose the same video cartoon to watch before bedtime. I asked for a referral to an occupational therapist or a behaviour therapist. Our paediatrician reminded me of Domenico's gender. Boys reach many developmental milestones later than girls. I went home, scared and feeling very alone. No referral.

After every appointment, I would describe the doctor's apparent apathy to Gian. His commitment to putting food on our table and paying our bills kept him on the job and out of the doctor's office. He took on the financial health of our entire family single-handedly. He even missed many of his own appointments with health care practitioners because of work responsibilities. But Gian was very present in the decision-making process and we shared a united frustration over what troubled me.

I returned, months later, with a request for a psychological assessment. This was my fourth attempt to get help for my son. Domenico's paediatrician finally made a referral to a developmental paediatrician. I felt like I had just won the lottery.

The developmental paediatrician I was referred to assessed Domenico in a robotic, almost sterile manner. It was unsettling. Domenico could not sit for any length of time. He could not focus long enough to complete any task, such as a puzzle or colouring activity. The developmental paediatrician asked me to hold Domenico down while she cornered him with the use of a small table. She placed a piece of paper and some crayons in front of him. She made observations and took notes as Domenico struggled.

I was then asked to leave the office. The developmental paediatrician wanted to gauge Domenico's reaction to my absence. She wanted to ascertain if Domenico would become upset if I left. She was looking for separation anxiety, and found none.

Every parent remembers their child's first day of school: the hugs, the tears, the promises that they would be reunited very soon. On Domenico's and Roberto's first days of Junior Kindergarten, I experienced extreme separation anxiety. Fear, actually. They were indifferent. On Roberto's first day of Senior Kindergarten, he looked in my direction as the school bus was pulling away from our home. He wasn't looking at me as if to say, "I'll miss you." He was looking through me. But I skipped my way up the driveway all the same, because he looked.

I guess the developmental paediatrician had seen enough. She bid us farewell and asked us to return in two months' time. At the second appointment, a diagnosis of autism was delivered. "Mrs. Sansalone, your son has autism: you know it and I know it." My son has autism and I knew it? But I didn't know.

I remember crying the entire drive home, sixty minutes of flood waters. I wasn't devastated; I was confused. My understanding of autism was skeletal at the time. The first thing I did when I returned home was call Gian who was out with our eighteen-month-old Roberto. I don't remember his reaction to the news and neither does he. I then called my parents. My dad answered the telephone. I relayed what the doctor had said. The deficiencies observed in Domenico's development were consistent with a diagnosis of autism. I told my father that I believed this to be true. I could see it now. Domenico had delays in his communication skills, he engaged in repetitive behaviours, and he did not form relationships. The last thing I said to my dad before hanging up was *I think it's serious.* I knew something was wrong. I knew my son needed help. But I thought everything was going to be okay.

Domenico was now almost four years of age. It had taken ten months to obtain a diagnosis. It had taken ten months to learn that the remainder of our lives was going to be anything but normal. We had lost ten months of early intervention strategies. Why did it have to take so long? I am not afraid of the truth. I am afraid of living in the darkness of ignorance.

Obtaining a diagnosis for Roberto was less formal, and almost incidental. "And, by the way, Mrs. Sansalone, your other son Roberto is also on the autism spectrum," was the unspoken conclusion from various health care providers who became involved with Domenico and then later Roberto. I brought Roberto to each and every one of Domenico's appointments to obtain services for speech, occupational, and behaviour therapy, as well as to gain access to community agencies. Anecdotal observations were being made by health care providers. We were all watching Roberto for the signs of autism, and it was plain as day.

Twenty years later, the diagnostic process has improved. Observations and consultations with parents and health care providers are required in order to make a diagnosis. Early signs of autism can be detected in infants as young as six to eighteen months. When a diagnosis is made, intervention can begin. The earlier, the better!

After confirming her initial impression of autism, the developmental paediatrician made many referrals – speech and language pathology, audiology, occupational therapy, behaviour therapy, Kerry's Place

Autism Services, and Geneva Centre for Autism, to name a few. She also made a referral to a doctor to study the genetics of autism.

This doctor's diagnostic process differed from the one I had just experienced. Both Domenico and Roberto were to be assessed at their first appointment. The doctor came to the three of us as we sat in the waiting room. He explained what we could expect. First, he wanted to visit with each of my sons individually. Two of his colleagues would be joining us. The doctor asked which of my sons should go first. Given Roberto's attention span, I chose him. And off he went with the doctor. Not more than five minutes later, Roberto emerged carrying a toy, happy and smiling. Next it was Domenico's turn. In just over five minutes, the doctor returned and invited me and Roberto to join Domenico and the others in his office.

A group discussion followed with a question and answer exchange. I had two questions. The first was about intervention strategies and treatment options. At that time, my research had concluded that there were two basic courses of action in helping those with autism. One was Applied Behaviour Analysis (ABA). The other was Social Communication Therapy. ABA aims to correct inappropriate and challenging behaviours by focusing on reinforcement of desirable behaviours. A commitment of approximately twenty to forty hours a week was mandatory. Social Communication Therapy involves placement of a child with autism in a setting with his or her peers who are developing normally, such as a preschool program. The principal objective is exposure to socially sanctioned means of communication, play skills, and behaviour. The child with autism, in time, would imitate and learn.

My second question was directed towards the suggestion of a secondary diagnosis. The presence of a developmental disability for both Domenico and Roberto was implied but never delivered, never documented in physician reports. I wanted to know if a developmental disability included cognition. The answer was yes. I should have known. Perhaps I needed time to fully process that this was not a death sentence.

The doctor provided a synopsis of the two main treatment plans available at the time. He said that if these were his children, he would enrol them in a preschool program. He would focus on the social and communication delays. He would not introduce ABA. He frowned on the practice of subjecting a young child to lengthy behavioural training sessions. The benefits were not worth it, in his opinion. The child could develop skills in a more natural and compassionate manner.

He gave me the affirmation I was looking for. I did not have the data nor the experience required to make an educated decision about which treatment approach to follow, so I followed my instincts. I did what felt right. With today's advances in autism research and the availability of social programming, I would have made a different decision for my sons. I would have introduced a balance between ABA and Social Communication Therapy. Today, with the World Wide Web at my fingertips, I would have known what to do.

Parents receiving a diagnosis of autism today are at an advantage with easy access to the Internet. They have the resources to learn about autism from the comforts of their home and in a timely manner. A greater number of treatment options are available for parents to research in order to make informed decisions. Twenty years ago, parents like me had to rely on books and articles. We had to attend workshops and consult with health care providers to learn about autism. We had to complete lengthy questionnaires. Our names had to go on waiting lists for services. When Roberto's name eventually made it to the top of one list, I had to sit down. I asked the caller to remind me of what service I had requested. It had been three years; I had forgotten. She informed me that it had to do with toileting. Roberto needed help with toileting. I thanked the caller but declined the six home visits that were being offered. I had already implemented strategies and we were making progress. Thanks all the same.

So much time has passed since receiving Domenico's diagnosis. I still remember the last time I saw the developmental paediatrician in January of 1996. After giving me the news, she handed me a pamphlet about autism. There was a beautiful little boy on the front cover. He was wearing a sailor's hat. Years later, I learned the boy's name and met his father at an information session for parents. I still have the pamphlet.

Lesson learned - When approaching a new situation, ask questions, do your homework, research with caution, filter the information, develop an action plan, execute your plan, make changes along the way as needed, never ever give up, and pray!

# Chapter Four

## AUTISM SPECTRUM DISORDER

*The word "autism" still conveys a fixed and dreadful meaning to most people—they visualize a child mute, rocking, screaming, inaccessible, cut off from human contact. And we almost always speak of autistic children, never of autistic adults, as if such children never grew up, or were somehow mysteriously spirited off the planet, out of society.*

**TEMPLE GRANDIN**

It has been suggested that people with an Autism Spectrum Disorder (ASD) live in their own world. That they avoid eye contact. That they resist human interaction. Can I invite you on a journey into the unknown? Allow me to take you through the labyrinth of the autistic mind. If at any time you want to hold my hand, please do, for this journey can be a little frightening and confusing. But it may not be so bad. We all have a little bit of autism in us.

Autism is defined by a triad of impairments: communication, socialization, and behaviour.

*Communication.* Every person on the spectrum struggles in the area of communication, ranging from verbal to non-verbal to somewhere in between. Many resist engaging in any form of reciprocal conversation because it is so difficult. For those who are verbal, some are limited to a form of speech known as echolalia. This repetition of words and sounds is based on a memorized pattern. Functional communication is therefore considered the main focus in giving those with autism a voice. They need to be taught that communication serves a purpose, such as requesting, rejecting or commenting.

Domenico developed a vocabulary of twenty words that were muted by the time of his third birthday. Some children with autism develop functional verbal communication up to the age of three at which time they begin to regress. Others, like Roberto, may demonstrate a deficiency in their language development in their first year of life.

Domenico *used* to count the stairs, "one, two, three, eight." My favourite memory of his pre-diagnostic years is of him running to the front door and saying, "shoes on." He was asking to go outside to play. For a child whose language is developing normally, this represents functional verbal communication. I wish I had recorded it, just to hear him speak again. Roberto has never spoken a word in his life. Domenico and Roberto remain non-verbal to this day.

For people with autism who are non-verbal like my sons, behaviour is considered an invaluable form of communication. In our efforts to understand what they may be trying to tell us, we observe their behaviours. Observations are subjective and thus susceptible to misinterpretation. Without confirmation from Domenico and Roberto, I do not always know with absolute certainty what they are trying to say. But making observations is all I have. So, over the years, I have learned to read Domenico's and Roberto's non-verbal forms of communication. Through their behaviours, gestures, facial expressions, and body language, they give me clues. This is how they tell me what they need or want. When a new or challenging behaviour presents itself without any warning, I first rule out any physiological explanation. Ear infections, sore throats, joint pains, headaches, and gastrointestinal discomfort - they feel it all.

Once the source of a new behaviour is identified, intervention can begin immediately. When illness or physiological processes have been ruled out and the all clear has been given by our primary care physician, I dig deeper. When Roberto resists putting on his shoes, I deduce he has a blister. When he tries to tame his wavy hair, I bring him for a haircut. He is telling me that he prefers his hair to be short. When he repeatedly brushes his chin strap, I shave it off. At times, his facial hair feels itchy to him. When Domenico dashes from the side window to the front door in anticipation of company arriving, I know he enjoys time with family and friends. When he rips the tags from his clothing, I understand his intolerance to labels. Some labels bother me too. Domenico and Roberto say so much, without uttering a single word.

Some behaviours have no communicative intent on behalf of the person with autism. They do not engage in these behaviours to relay a need or a want. The motivation behind the behaviour is not to initiate a social exchange. These behaviours are non-functional in that they appear senseless to us, but they have significance to the person with autism. They are consistent with the core diagnostic feature of ASD (compulsions, rituals, limited interests, and insistence on sameness). They support the person's need to engage in stereotypical movements and repetitive manipulation of objects. They speak to a commonly observed adherence to routine and resistance to change. Domenico in particular has an endless barrage of non-functional behaviours. He will do something that follows no logical clarity of thought, but for Domenico, it makes perfect sense. His entire day unfolds like a well-scripted play, only he is not acting.

Many of Domenico's non-functional behaviours communicate his need for predictability. Drop in at any time of the day and I will bring you up to speed. If you are a morning person, come early; this conversation begins the minute he welcomes the day. Every morning, he will squeeze my hand as we pray "Grace before Meals" at the breakfast table. While dressing, he will knock the toothbrushes over and then straighten them up again. He will then come to me to apply his acne cream and clean the lenses of his glasses. Together, we walk downstairs where he will disassemble his tubes (I will explain later) and lay them to rest until his return. I extend a cardboard barrier across the bathroom door so he does not walk in as Rocco showers (he learned how to unlock the door). Domenico will then proceed to sit on Rocco's bed, open and close the drawer of his end table several times, and vocalize. Not sure how long you are planning on staying, but it is not even eight o'clock in the morning.

*Socialization.* Conventional wisdom supports the assumption that people with autism remain detached from society by choice. I disagree. The differences in how they perceive social information and navigate the fluctuating nuances inherent in human interactions present real barriers to developing meaningful relationships. Reciprocity as the basis for all social interactions also presents a challenge for people with autism, irrespective of their social functioning and communication abilities. Both Domenico and Roberto respond positively to an act of friendship. But they need help relating to others. They need help developing socially sanctioned behaviours.

Some of Domenico's and Roberto's behaviours may be considered awkward or inappropriate in a social setting. Domenico may barge in on another person's personal space. He needs reminders to knock before opening a closed door and entering the room. For him, my morning mouthwash rinse is a spectator sport. Sometimes I cannot see what I am writing because his head is in the way (he gets that close). When visiting a new place, Domenico will walk into every single room and open drawers and closets for a thorough orientation. This ritual is carried out even when returning to a familiar location.

Something may have changed, and Domenico needs to know. Roberto will only join a social circle if invited. Once there, the encounter needs to be brief and animated. He will return to his comfort zone the minute your back is turned. When entering any waiting room or familiar setting, Roberto will walk over to the same chair, every single time. If someone is sitting in that chair, Roberto will stand and wait, until the kind stranger moves. He displays a similar behaviour at the public hot tub he frequents. Roberto will nudge his way closer and closer to a fellow guest who may be sitting in his spot. Eventually, the new friend makes way for Roberto.

Establishing boundaries is a fundamental social skill that Domenico and Roberto both need to develop. Making inferences and understanding social cues is another area that requires intervention. People with autism may not understand humour, sarcasm, or emotion but rather take your word at face value. "I am so hungry I could eat a horse" is an idiom commonly used without any thought of what it literally means. A phrase like this could cause the following reaction from a person with autism: "That's crazy talk; you are supposed to ride a horse, not eat it." If you tell someone on the autism spectrum that "I am dying of heat," those who are capable might dial 911 in a panic, begging you to hang on until help arrives. You may be feeling a little melancholy, but unless Niagara Falls is gushing from each eye, a person with autism may not even notice your somber mood.

People on the autism spectrum are at risk of living a marginalized existence, of not being accepted into social circles because of their impairments. If they are not taught how to integrate into society, they will simply live from the outside, looking in.

I have an image of Roberto etched with indelible ink in my memory. It was before I knew he had autism. He was just a toddler at the time. I wish I could erase it, but then why would I? As I drove up to the daycare at the end of my work day, I saw Roberto pacing back and forth by the perimeter of the outdoor enclosed area. All the other children were doing what came so naturally to them: they were playing. I wanted to close my eyes and immediately die. I promised myself right then and there that my son was not going to live his life on the sidelines. Shoulder to shoulder, we would find our way; we would build a bridge.

*Behaviour.* People with autism share a need to establish patterns of behaviour that are repetitive in nature. There is a predictability and routine within these patterns. An association to a person, place, or object is often attached to a behaviour.

At our dinner table, Domenico will stomp his feet several times while eating his salad, every night. At your dinner table, he will not stomp his feet, even if you serve him salad. Some behaviours are transferable to new locations and new people, while some are specific. Other behaviours are rigid, making it difficult to change a behaviour that is inappropriate.

Roberto does not like clutter. It creates confusion in his mind. "My brain is the only place I have to live; keep it neat and tidy," Roberto pleads. The soap dispenser in the washroom cannot remain on the counter; it must vanish, out of sight, out of mind, into the cabinet when not in use. This behaviour is specific to the washroom he uses. Roberto only uses one of the three washrooms in our home. The soap dispensers in the other two washrooms can remain on the counter, but they must hug the faucet.

Each evening after dinner, Domenico will go into the kitchen drawer, take two elastics from the bunch, break them, and then discard both. After drying his hands, each and every time, Roberto will remove the towel from his washroom and tuck it far back into the linen closet. He will then proceed to our second washroom and remove that towel. Into the linen closet you go; Roberto's orders. Domenico and Roberto give the term "creature of habit" an entirely different dimension.

Over their lifetime, some behaviours will be replaced with new ones. Some behaviours will remain a part of their daily routine. Domenico leaves his drink until the end of every meal, and then he empties his glass in one breath. Always has, and in all likelihood, always will. He crumbles the crust of his toast at breakfast. The more crumbs, the better. This behaviour dates back to as far as my memory takes me. Roberto used to stand in one place in our home upon his return from elementary school. He would jump and jump and jump until dinner was served. When we purchased a glider for him, he found security and relaxation in his new place. The jumping stopped, thankfully, as he had been damaging his hips from all that jumping. In elementary school, during recess, Roberto would go to the same area of the playground and not move. Wherever he goes, Roberto finds a comfort zone. Always has, and in all likelihood, always will. While waiting to enter his elementary school in the mornings, Domenico used to rub his backpack against the brick exterior of the building. When he began secondary school, this behaviour ended. It had been specific to the morning routine of waiting outside his elementary school. In secondary school, Domenico entered the building upon arrival, no waiting, no idle time, no rubbing. Roberto developed an intolerance of buttons on his clothing. No shirt is safe, no pant protected. Roberto even pulls the buttons off his father's clothing. When I lock Gian's clothing in the armoire, I feel that I am harbouring a fugitive. I sew the waistband of Roberto's pants to close it in place of a button. Both Domenico and Roberto pull their jacket zippers all the way up. To them, this is logical. The zipper is there to be used. These types of behaviours underscore the pervasive nature of autism.

Attachment to objects is also prevalent in those with autism. Domenico carries tubes that he connects and manipulates into different shapes of his making. They are plastic, accordion-like, and hollow and Domenico loves them. In essence, they are an extension of him. Roberto carries a cologne bottle with him. He never uses it, never smells it but finds comfort in having it close by.

Transitions are challenging for people on the autism spectrum, and some transitions are more challenging than others. Their fear of moving through these changes could manifest as perplexing behaviours. Imagine for a minute how you felt when you attended a different school, moved into a new house, accepted a promotion at work, married your best friend, started a family, or purchased your first vehicle. No doubt you experienced some degree of anxiety, even if the change was positive and progressive. Now imagine a person with autism who has impairments in all three areas of the triad. Imagine Roberto. He, in particular, has extreme difficulty with transitions, even within a given day. Roberto will sprint from his comfort zone to the washroom when called for bath time. He may even walk through you if you happen to be on his path. Moving from point A to point B is terrifying for Roberto at times, even in the security and familiarity of his own home. Adapting to winter after autumn, what's the big deal? It is a big deal for Roberto, every year. He now has to wear his winter jacket. Roberto walks out of the house wearing his jacket, toque, and mitts. But once in the school bus, Roberto removes his jacket. His toque and mitts stay on. He does the same during the ride home from school. Even when the mercury plummets to -35°C, Roberto will not keep his jacket on when riding the bus. Domenico and Roberto will continue to require support as they grow through countless transitions in their lives.

There is often an underlying causative factor behind autistic behaviours, such as a communicative attempt or a coping mechanism. Identifying the reason for the behaviour will contribute to an effective intervention strategy and a greater quality of life.

Assumptions, Autism, and Aggression. Before going any further, can we talk about this? An automatic assumption that autism and aggression go hand in hand is often made. Please do not go there. Please do not believe that people with autism are aggressive by virtue of their diagnosis. The behaviours demonstrated by a person with autism are as normal as that of any child, adolescent or adult at a given time in his or her development. For the autistic population however, less tolerance is given and preconceptions are made. Imagine for a moment the inherent anxiety of living with autism. The degree of impairments and the level of support are contributing factors to the a person's tendency to escalate. Can you blame them, especially those who are non-verbal? Behaviour is communication. What other means do they have to relay anxiety, confusion, depression, fear, frustration, loneliness, pain, sadness, and any other stimuli that you and I may feel at different times in our lives? They experience these emotions, just as we do! However, unlike you and me, they have limited means of communicating and understanding those feelings and impetuses. And they may feel them with greater intensity. Sometimes even a positive emotion like happiness becomes challenging due to self-regulation. Domenico becomes very vocal and energetic, all day long, when content.

I remember one technician's automatic response when she learned Domenico has autism and needed blood work completed. She immediately offered to call a colleague to help hold Domenico down during the procedure. She concluded that, because he is on the spectrum, he would be uncooperative and combative. She did not know Domenico. I had come prepared with a visual for Domenico to look at while his blood was being drawn. It was an actual photograph of blood being drawn from a vein in his arm. I used the visual aid to "talk" to him about what was about to happen while waiting for our turn. He was watching his favourite cartoon on his portable DVD player while waiting and would continue to do so as a distraction. Finally, I was there to offer any support needed. I assured her that she could proceed; we were prepared. She was delighted and surprised at the ease in which two vials of blood were drawn. I was delighted and proud, and was actually beaming.

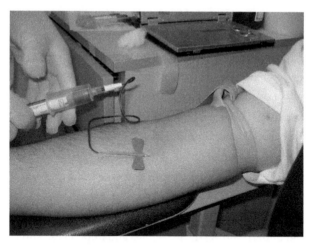

Build for me a visual world

Both Domenico and Roberto have engaged in behaviours that may be perceived as aggression. Domenico bit the arm of a family member when he was four years old. He was being physically restrained at the time in a chokehold. This roughhousing was all in good fun, but Domenico did not know that. Later in grade one, he was also restrained. As a defence mechanism, he tried to bite his teacher. Since that time, Domenico has never bitten another person. Roberto demonstrates self-injurious behaviours such as head-banging and hitting his chin but only when he is extremely agitated. Parental consent (from yours truly) for two educators to enter the washroom with Domenico at school (the only time he is not supervised) finally led to an explanation for the bruising Domenico had on his left hip. After washing his hands, he would thrust his hip against the sink. One night, Domenico kicked a hole in the ceiling of his bedroom while lying on the top bunk bed. He was hungry. When Domenico is anxious, he will stomp his feet, slam doors and drawers, and vocalize, with a scowl on his face. Roberto, one idle Monday afternoon, plucked his eyebrows off with his own hands. He was quick and thorough. It was a snow day, there was no school, and this was a change. Domenico pulls his toenails off when he is restless and cannot settle to sleep, usually on a Sunday evening.

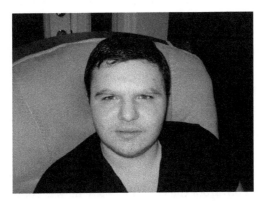

Idle hands governed by the autistic mind

Please get to know someone with autism before passing judgement. Please spend some time with them before making a correlation between autism and aggression. You may be as pleasantly surprised as the technician.

Sensory Processing Disorder (SPD) and Obsessive Compulsive Disorder (OCD), although not qualifying characteristics for a diagnosis of autism, are common in ASD. Domenico and Roberto, to varying degrees, demonstrate behaviours consistent with both disorders.

*Sensory Processing Disorder.* People on the autism spectrum have impairments in their brain's ability to respond to stimuli from their body's basic sensory systems. These sensory systems are responsible for identifying and processing sights, sounds, smells, tastes, temperature, pain, and the position and movement of the body.

Roberto has demonstrated feeding problems from infancy to date because of SPD. He discriminated amongst food textures and feeding items very early on, discarding his bottle of milk for his cup of juice by age two. I became known at my grocery store as the "Strawberry

Lady" because, at one point, that was the only fruit Roberto would eat. I purchased strawberries in abundance, but I could not find a utensil that Roberto would tolerate in my efforts to teach him to feed himself.

My occupational therapist made house calls and had a plan. She set things up for success by coming into Roberto's comfort zone: his home. Her timing was also by design, as she arrived at lunch time when Roberto was very motivated by food. I had prepared his favourite meal: bite-sized pasta noodles in tomato sauce. She offered him one noodle at a time. *Brilliant*, I thought, but I had my doubts. She secured one noodle on the end of the cup and had him take the noodle by mouth from the cup. She knew he was comfortable with the feel of his cup because he already drank his juice from it independently. She repeated this several times. Then, wait for it, she put the next noodle on a fork, and brought the noodle, fork, and cup to his mouth together. The fork sat just below the cup, out of sight. Success: he took the noodle from the fork! She repeated this several times. Then, she used the fork only. Success again, but it did not stop there. The best part was when she put the noodle on the fork and placed it in front of him. You guessed it! He picked up the fork and fed himself. Roberto learned to use a fork that afternoon. He finally learned to feed himself. I was on such a spiritual high, I thought I could fly!

Toileting a person with an ASD is more complicated than toileting a typically developing child. Roberto's toileting difficulties can also be attributed to Sensory Processing Disorder. His toileting was accomplished over a thirteen-year period. Roberto had great success during the day but overnight, he wore a pull-up. One night stands out as a defining moment. I started to put on Roberto's pull-up as per usual. The look of embarrassment that replaced his ready smile reduced me to tears. *That was it*, I decided, *no more pull-up*. For the next two years, I set my alarm for two a.m. I would wake Roberto to use the washroom, and then back to our respective beds we went. Most mornings he woke up dry, but some mornings he needed a bath. *I will stay up all night, Roberto; I will never sleep again if that is what it takes to never see that look again.*

Toileting continues to present a challenge for Roberto. The sensation of emptying his bladder and bowels is very uncomfortable for him. He will sit on the toilet for up to an hour to avoid the feeling. Sometimes, he doesn't even feel or recognize the natural impulses that his body sends, telling him he needs to void. I sought advice from a behaviour therapist. Two hundred and forty dollars later, I have a strategy that is effective. *Ouch, that hurt. My bank account is probably suffering from acute withdrawal syndrome.* The intervention utilizes the concept of time with the aid of a Time Timer. The Time Timer looks like a clock and has a red dial that can be set for up to one hour. The red dial illustrates time elapsing. Every morning when Roberto enters the washroom, I set the Time Timer to fifteen minutes and then I give him privacy. Once that time has elapsed, the Time Timer beeps and I return. Sometimes I massage his forehead to help him relax and verbally prompt him. Ninety percent of the time, nothing. We move on to washing his face; putting on his deodorant, shirt, and acne cream; and then he tries again. The Time Timer is set for another fifteen-minute interval. Eighty percent of the time, success. Roberto then independently finishes dressing and washes his hands. Try this technique. I am giving it to you free of charge, and it works!

*Obsessive Compulsive Disorder.* Intrusive, unwanted, recurrent, and persistent thoughts, images, feelings, ideas, or impulses can potentially debilitate those afflicted with this anxiety disorder. The compulsive tendencies of these obsessions quite literally imprison someone in his or her own mind. They simply cannot find the "off" button.

Domenico and Roberto both suffer from OCD. Domenico smothers one family member in particular with hugs and kisses every time he sees her (I like this obsession). Roberto will wipe the sink bone-dry after every use. He will adjust and reposition the couch pillows several times a day. *I prefer that the pillows rest comfortably on their sides, but if you insist they stand at attention, I salute you Roberto; that's fine by me.* Domenico and Roberto share a long history of skin abrasions that become infected. They will perseverate on a minor injury such as a superficial scrape. Many years ago, within a month of each other Domenico and Jennifer sustained similar trauma due to a fall. Jennifer's wound healed in one week. Domenico's healed in six months and required two rounds of oral antibiotics. He continuously picked at the sore. Every time we visit his general practitioner, Domenico has to make sure all their calendars are flipped to the correct month. His obsession with hangers got out of hand over a two-year period of time. I could not make heads or tails of the behaviour. But it involved wanting to see two hangers in his closet remain bare and ripping shirts in order to achieve this. The only pattern I observed was the days of the week he was most likely to become concerned about the hangers. Saturday morning, the start of the weekend and Monday morning, the start of a new week had me standing at the ready. As a final attempt to correct this habit, I imposed consequences, making him wear the ripped shirt at home only. The behaviour continued. One Monday morning, ten minutes before his bus was scheduled to pick him up, Domenico ripped the shirt he was wearing. I sewed it while on his person and made him wear it to his day program. I created a visual of him wearing the ripped shirt and superimposed the universal symbol of "no" over it (red circle with a diagonal line). Success, finally, but every now and then, Domenico asks me if he can remove a shirt (walking towards his bedroom, pointing, vocalizing). I point to the picture taped to the inside door of his closet door, say "no", and walk away. Roberto will open each and every door on the main floor of the house, all the way please, with the exception of his washroom door, which must stay closed. All the doors in the basement must also remain closed. He rearranges and stacks items in the refrigerator, leaving shelves completely empty. You get the idea. The list goes on and on. And it changes.

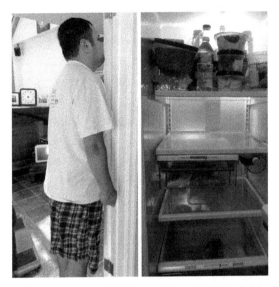

Roberto and what SPD (Page 49) and OCD look like

Roberto was not always preoccupied with the location and placement of items in the house. New obsessions simply surfaced. No magazines on the coffee table. Shoes must be in the closet, with laces undone. No kitchen utensils in the sink. No clothes on the suit stand. Tissues must be tucked in the Kleenex box, television remote controls must be aligned, small pieces of furniture must be flush against the wall, countertop objects must be corralled in the corner, bananas must be separated from the bunch, and so on. Roberto's compulsions seem to come and go virtually overnight. One day, a pair of shorts went missing from where they hung on the suit stand in my bedroom. I knew Roberto had removed them. He is the only one in the family who tidies up. *Thanks for the help, Pal.* If I was to find the shorts, I had to think like Roberto. I had to see the world through the lens of the autistic eye. Years of observation had taught me that obsessions tend to be repetitive in nature and thus predictable. With this conclusion, I devised a plan to recover the shorts. The next day, I implemented my plan. After Roberto left for school, I hung a second pair of shorts on the suit stand. I anticipated that Roberto would remove this pair just as he had removed the other. I had watched him in action so many times, I was able to identify when he would be most inclined to commit the crime. Roberto's obsessions woke up again once he was home from school. If he was to remove the shorts, he would do it then. My plan put me in close proximity to my bedroom. From that vantage point, I could witness the shorts' abduction. I had a hunch that Roberto would put the second pair of shorts with the missing pair. This experiment could work. It was show time. Roberto returned from school and wasted no time. He noticed the shorts. I pretended to be engaged in my own task, oblivious to what he was doing in the next room. Roberto, unassuming, proceeded to remove the second pair of shorts from the suit stand and tuck them into the only drawer I had not checked. Eureka, there lay the first pair of shorts. It actually worked. My plan led me to the shorts and to a better understanding of his obsessions. Roberto becomes visually over-stimulated if his environment is crowded and untidy. Seeing clothing out of the drawers contributed to his uneasiness. He never went back to check if the shorts were still in the drawer. Roberto just wanted an uncluttered living space. For me, this exercise was another learning opportunity. Another window into the autistic mind. Another mystery solved. Just call me Sherlock, as in the detective!

Although there are commonalities amongst people with autism, there remains great variance in the severity and manifestation of the three impairments. My survival guide, above all, insists I stay the course and maintain predictability within a well-established routine. But when it comes to living with autism, I do not want to simply survive, I want to triumph. With sights set high, I keep a well-stocked medicine cabinet. What's in my medicine cabinet? So glad you asked.

Lesson learned - Autism is a puzzle to be understood and solved, not feared or dismissed, not pushed to the side.

# Chapter Five

## TAKE YOUR MEDICINE - IT WILL MAKE YOU FEEL BETTER

*A story - a true story - can heal as much as medicine can.*

**EBEN ALEXANDER**

Antipsychotics, antidepressants, anti-anxiety - give him something to keep him calm, help him sleep, improve his attention span, make it go away - PLEASE! There is no known cure for autism. There is no magic potion, no miracle drug to make him talk, make him social, make him behave. Medications prescribed to people with an ASD treat medical and behavioural conditions associated with autism; they do not treat autism. The core symptoms of autism (communication difficulties, social struggles, and repetitive behaviours) will not go away with the use of prescription and non-prescription medication. Anxiety, depression, attention deficit/hyperactivity disorder, gastrointestinal problems, sleep disturbances, and epilepsy are common amongst those with autism. Treating these conditions, together with educational approaches and behavioural therapy, is thought to promote the greatest quality of life.

The years have watered down my memory when it comes to medication. I do not remember making the decision to introduce mood-altering drugs to Domenico and Roberto. It just seemed to happen, as if mandatory. What was there to talk about; they needed medication, right? The answer is yes. They did need medication. Not everyone on the autism spectrum requires medication, but my sons do. In fact, they cannot function without it.

Roberto, who is younger, was prescribed medication before Domenico. He was eight years of age. It was 2002. Roberto's attention span was five minutes on a good day. He could not sit for any significant length of time. I had to do cartwheels to get Roberto to sleep, and when he eventually did, it felt more like a power nap. Roberto was just a little boy but already needed medication, as he probably would for life. It was a hard pill for this parent to swallow. But for Roberto, it was easy. He did not even need water to take one of his pills - gulp and the medicine went down. One parent pointed out my good fortune in Roberto taking his medication without coercion. I failed to see the blessing in my eight-year-old son having to take antipsychotics. I was just grateful that the medication took the edge off. By improving his ability to remain calm and focused, we could work on developing skills for life. Domenico would get by without medication until secondary school. He was thirteen years of age when medication was first prescribed. I had a feeling that this was only the beginning.

*Prescription medication.* Domenico has been on medication for ten years, Roberto for thirteen. Domenico and Roberto each take an antipsychotic to abate their irritability, an antidepressant to quiet their obsessive-compulsive tendencies, and seizure medication to control their epilepsy. Domenico was fifteen when he started having seizures. His paediatric neurologist prescribed Divalproex. Every time Domenico would have a seizure, the dosage of his seizure medication would increase. Roberto was almost eighteen before he had his first seizure. By that time, Domenico was under the care of a neurologist for adults. This neurologist took Roberto on as a new client but prescribed Clobazam, a different seizure medication. For a period of time, Domenico and Roberto were both taking the same dosage of Risperdal (antipsychotic) and Zoloft (antidepressant). One day, that all changed.

Roberto, more so than Domenico, has a greater sensitivity to medication. When he was twelve, Roberto demonstrated regressive behaviours. He was climbing furniture, not sleeping, and not eating. He was sitting cross-legged and putting his arms inside his sleeves. He would giggle senselessly in one breath and sob inconsolably in the next. We increased his daily dosage of Risperdal. It was 2006. Roberto showed improvements in his behaviour with this higher dosage. No further medication changes were necessary. We coasted for the next six years of *relative* ease, naive to the storm of 2013-2015. That storm almost capsized our lives.

It started in June of 2013. In response to restlessness and increased episodes of escalating agitation, we increased Roberto's daily dosage of Risperdal, one tablet at a time. After a lengthy trial and error period without the desired response, we replaced Risperdal with Abilify. It was now April of 2014. Abilify is also an antipsychotic. Roberto was not in distress while on Abilify, but he was in a constant state of heightened awareness. He was loud and vocal all day long, laughing at nothing. This went on for months on end. By the eighth month, it was evident that Abilify was the wrong medication for Roberto. We discontinued it and started Olanzapine in November of the same year. Olanzapine, relatively new, is classified as an atypical antipsychotic, how comforting. There was a honeymoon period. Initially, Roberto seemed to benefit from Olanzapine. He was relaxed, eating well, and following routines. One of the side effects of Olanzapine is drowsiness. Roberto was exhausted all the time, putting his head down on his desk at school and falling asleep in the bathtub at home. He even slept through a haircut. He looked over-medicated. I tried not to look. This was a side effect. I took it at face value. I reassured myself that his extreme fatigue would subside in time. And it did, but so did his ability to remain calm. I tried to remain optimistic as Roberto ran laps around the house. He was rubbing his abdomen all day long. He was awake all night long. In addition to drowsiness, difficulty with bowel movements while taking Olanzapine is another unfavourable possibility. Roberto would spend hours in the washroom with no success. Constipation was thought to be the root cause of the rubbing and insomnia. A stool softener was recommended. Once we determined how much Roberto needed to take, regular bowel movements returned. Roberto, however, was still pacing the house, day and night, though he was not rubbing his abdomen. He was also having weekly bowel accidents due to the soft stool. The adverse effects of this third medication cancelled the benefits. Over a period of five days, we reduced the daily dosage of Olanzapine to zero. By day five, Roberto had returned to a calm, alert state. He was sleeping through the night, eating well, having good days at school, and seemed happy, with no pacing. On day six, I was to start Roberto on a fourth antipsychotic, Quetiapine. I prepared his medication for the next day but when morning came, I could not bring myself to give it to him. For the next eight days, Roberto did not take anything for irritability. I actually entertained the idea that Roberto no longer needed medication (a Hail Mary moment). Roberto had been on antipsychotic medication for twelve years. I had thought this would continue for life. I was waiting for the world to come to an end, because this was too good to be true. And it did; our world did come crashing down. It was too good to be true. Everything went sideways. Roberto became extremely unsettled. Autism was just too much for him to handle. I had to feed him and prevent him from hurting himself, but when I looked into his eyes, I saw a void. Roberto was lost to himself and to his family. The situation became grave. He desperately needed help. He desperately needed the medication. I gave him the pill. As the fourth antipsychotic, it was also atypical, also ineffective. Roberto was sleeping the night while on Quetiapine but his awake time was a nightmare. He would hold both his bladder and bowels for up to twenty-four hours. He wandered aimlessly, stared at the wall, and had to be fed. It was hard to stay positive. I was losing hope. I was starting to shut down as a human being. The emotional pain was overwhelming. Convinced that Roberto was suffering from the side effects of Quetiapine, Risperdal was reintroduced. This was the same medication Roberto had been on since the age of eight. It was May of 2015. We had come full circle but added Lorazepam, an anti-anxiety medication. For the first week, I held my breath, waiting for the ground to give way from beneath my feet. For the second week, I held my breath, waiting for regressive behaviours to resurface. By week three, I exhaled a cautious sigh of relief. It was a new day.

In Domenico's case, the introduction of mood stabilizing drugs helped him cope with significant life transitions. Moving from elementary to secondary school and then secondary school to adult day programming seemed to necessitate the aid of medication. The inherent hormonal changes, insecurity, anxiety, and confusion that accompany adolescence threatened to exclude Domenico from educational opportunities. He was prescribed Risperdal and Zoloft when he was in grade nine. Domenico then enjoyed seven successful years of secondary school. Day programming presented many changes (we talk about day programming in Chapters 9 and 10). To help him manage his heightened agitation we substituted Risperdal for Abilify in September of 2014. Domenico did not respond positively to Abilify. His central nervous system was set to overdrive. He was in constant motion and very vocal. In November of 2014, we changed to Olanzapine. Olanzapine offers a sedative effect which Domenico needed. He responded favourably to Olanzapine with the absence of any adverse effects. The same medication that had compromised Roberto's well-being benefitted Domenico. How can two brothers, who share the same genetic material, living under the same roof, and presenting with the same disorder, be so different? I asked myself the same question.

With medication, there is always a risk-benefit consideration that goes into the decision-making process. What may help one person could potentially cause harmful side effects to another. The same medication can be prescribed for more than one condition. Divalproex, prescribed for management of seizures, also helps with mood stabilization. It was prescribed to Domenico for his seizures but may have a secondary benefit of helping him remain calm. Determining the correct dosage of the medication prescribed is imperative in receiving the maximum benefit from the drug. It is a heart-wrenching experience, more complex than I had imagined. And my imagination sometimes takes me where I do not want to go.

I have a recurrent, waking nightmare. Every evening, as I shampoo Roberto's hair, I run my fingers over the swelling on his forehead and I remember all the times he has head-banged over his lifetime. Consequently, the bump is permanent. As I massage the shampoo through his wavy hair, I visualize an anxious Roberto succumb to a self-inflicted, fatal blow. He hits his head so hard against the kitchen window that shards of glass embed his skull and drain the life blood out of him. This moment of dread is brief but raw. The thought is diluted once I start rinsing the shampoo out of Roberto's hair. I then finish bathing him and move on, knowing that tomorrow it will all come back again. Will there ever be a pill to stop Roberto from head-banging?

I never thought it would be so difficult to determine which medication and how much of that medication would be required to give Domenico and Roberto a chance at life. I have always had confidence in the medical profession and always will. The storm of 2013-2015 taught me that I had to be a part of that confidence. I had to be involved in the decision-making. I had to keep learning.

*Non-prescription medication.* I never experimented when it came to Domenico and Roberto. I believe in the science of conventional medicine. When I lived through the negative side effects of some prescription medications, I considered alternative medicine. At a minimum, I had a responsibility to Domenico and Roberto to ask the questions. I consulted with a naturopathic doctor for Roberto primarily. After gathering information to develop a profile, she recommended five different supplements. Specifically, her list included a probiotic, fish oil, vitamin B-complex, vitamin D, and a mood supplement. I was prepared to introduce only one supplement at a time. In this way, I could determine if any improvement or detriment was directly related to the supplement. When I asked her which one of the five I should consider first, she recommended the probiotic. There would be no risk of contraindications while taking the probiotic, she assured me. It would help restore the good flora in the gut, she explained, which was often compromised when taking medication for extended periods of time. No harm would come. I had to give it a try. I owed it to my son. She also cautioned me to limit or completely eliminate wheat, sugar, and dairy from Roberto's diet while increasing his water consumption. I put the brakes on. Any change would be gradual and after careful consideration. I could not demand so much of Roberto all at once. I went with the probiotic. Roberto swallowed the white powder effortlessly, indifferent to its function. No improvement was observed but it had only been a few months. I was confident it would help with his digestive health. I also started Domenico on the same probiotic. But I had to stop, not because the results were ambiguous and not because it was an additional responsibility for me. I stopped because the money ran out.

I am not a doctor, pharmacist, therapist, naturopath, or scientist. I do not have a working knowledge of medication. How was I to make a decision about prescription or non-prescription medication as a viable treatment option for my sons? I could start by asking questions, and I did. I asked countless questions to every health care provider involved in my sons' care. This exercise resulted in a proliferation of conflicting information. Rather than becoming frustrated, I collected and filtered the data obtained. I came to understand that the best way to find the answers is to live through the questions. I worked closely with my doctor, sending e-mail updates of Domenico's and Roberto's responses to new medication. I learned that people respond differently to the same medication, even when there is so much in common. I learned that a therapeutic level had to be reached before the benefits of some medication were realized. I completed several internet searches. In order to exercise independent judgement, I made a commitment to self-learning. I promised Domenico and Roberto that I would see them through any medication changes. We would work through the side effects together. I vowed to remain steadfast until I found a way. Twenty-five years later, it feels that I am just getting started.

Treating autism with medication is as pervasive as the disorder itself. There is no short-term remedy for this lifelong condition. Some days are harder than others. Sometimes, autism is a hard pill to swallow. Sometimes, I am deeply frightened. I want everything to go dark. Quitting, however, is never an option. I may not be able to do everything, but there is a lot I can do to enhance Domenico's and Roberto's lives. I have to believe that. Medication is only part of the solution. I know there are alternatives. I just have to find them. Come with me. But first, let's get some courage from the medicine cabinet. We are going to therapy.

Lesson learned - Stock your medicine cabinet with independent learning, unbiased judgment, collaborative effort, endurance, faith, courage, hope, and an abundance of love. When considering medication, start by educating yourself. Ask questions, work closely with your health care provider, study your options, do your homework - pray!

# Chapter Six

## A LIST AS LONG AS YOUR ARM
### Therapy

---

*I hear things more loudly. I see things more clearly.*
*I smell things more strongly. I feel things you*
*don't. I taste things differently. I have autism.*

---

**UNKNOWN**

As discussed in the last chapter, medical management of autism's core symptoms underscores the notion that there is no "take two pills and call me in the morning" express resolution. Non-medical management is equally complex. No single treatment will be effective for every person on the spectrum. An internet search will produce a list of treatment options as long as your arm. Developing a treatment plan can be intimidating. Where do you go for services, how long is the waiting list, how many hours a week are involved, how much will it cost? These are some of the questions parents face. When I was starting out, the list of treatment options was less than impressive. Integrated services that would be delivered under one roof did not exist. With today's advances, there are a greater number of treatments available. The short list could include play, art, music, and animal-assisted therapy; applied behaviour analysis; as well as behavioural, occupational, and speech therapy. My list of treatment options for Domenico and Roberto was much shorter. The diagnosing doctor made referrals for behavioural, occupational, and speech therapy. The waiting lists to obtain government funded services were illogical. I had to dig deep into my empty pockets in order to access the private sector for therapy. This translated to a shrinking bank account with overdraft protection (and premature grey hair). No savings for Rocco's and Jennifer's future, no retirement package. All the therapy that Domenico and Roberto have received to date has been paid for out of pocket. With that said, let's go to therapy.

*Behaviour Therapy.* Behaviour therapists often take on the role of consultants. They come into a setting and make observations about the environment, the activities, and the person who needs help. Once enough data has been collected about what triggers or calms challenging behaviours, suggestions are made. Intervention strategies are then considered. A trial and error period follows as strategies are implemented. Troubleshooting continues until the difficult behaviours have been corrected. That is the Coles Notes version of how behaviour therapy works.

This is my version. I sought the advice of a behaviour therapist for a subject matter that is completely natural, very common, extremely sensitive, and potentially problematic if not addressed. I will not keep you in suspense. It is the "M" word: masturbation. There, I said it. It was hard, but I said it. Did I just use the word hard? Happy coincidence. If you need a moment before we go any further, I will wait with you. My uneasiness and reservation about this topic had to go away (easier said than done). I remember hearing a story about masturbation training that disturbed me. A man with non-verbal autism was extremely frustrated because the group home he lived in did not believe in the practice of masturbation on any account. Expected to bury these natural impulses forever, this young fellow resorted to problematic behaviour (self-harm, screaming) to get his point across,

to be heard. His parents had renounced their rights to make decisions on his behalf. He was trapped in his own body. The hardship
his guardians imposed on him was preventable and inexcusable in my
humble opinion. I do not agree with denying someone the freedom
to be human. Domenico needed to learn that there was a time and a
place to masturbate. His inappropriate social behaviour was especially
prevalent at public swimming pools. I had to do something.

My first appointment with the behaviour therapist ended in homework being assigned. I had to read a book with an accompanying
video. If I could have read that book with my eyes closed, I would
have. I never did watch the video. Gian approached the matter from
an analytical perspective. He questioned the probability of creating
a breeding ground for new behaviours to develop by introducing
masturbation training. I agreed with him. I was not ready to implement any of the suggestions made in the reading. Instead, I redirected
Domenico's focus any time he was in a swimming pool. I kept him
engaged in different activities for the entire swim time. I know what
you are thinking: "You are a coward, Mirian." Right? You are right.
It was a Band-Aid solution that proved effective for the short-term.
I knew that eventually I would need a long-term plan. Years later, I
returned for a second appointment. Did I mention that the therapist
was a man? *The therapist was a man.* Go ahead and laugh; I did. But
I left that appointment with a course of action. Domenico would be
taught how, when, and where to masturbate. The number of training
sessions would depend on Domenico's learning curve. The therapist
would come to our house to teach Domenico. Once the objective
of this intervention was met, Domenico would *never* see this therapist *ever again in his lifetime*. That was key. Again, I was not ready. I
procrastinated. Short of laying an egg, I was behaving like a chicken.
(Humour is great therapy, and I had to laugh my way through this
uncomfortable space.) While I allowed the idea of masturbation
training to marinate, Domenico inherently learned over time while

showering. There have been no further concerns in this area since that time.

Then Roberto started demonstrating inappropriate behaviour on his first day at Program H. I met with the same behaviour therapist to discuss a plan of action. That plan would simmer until it had to be served. The initial behaviour of touching his private parts in public stopped as Roberto became familiar with the new program, new people, and new routine (the behaviour ended as his anxiety abated). Two months later, the behaviour returned. Remember the chicken from the earlier years? The one who considered masturbation training? She grew balls. I made an appointment. I sat down face to face with the male behaviour therapist and told him that I wanted him to teach Roberto how to masturbate. It was the first thing I said after hello. We came up with a plan. First, I was to purchase a masturbation tool. When I went online to purchase the item, the website prompted me to confirm that I was older than eighteen years of age. I felt dirty, like I was doing something wrong. But one's sexuality is not dirty; it is natural. Should Roberto demonstrate the need to masturbate, I would offer this tool to him. If he could learn its function and receive gratification, the job was done. Failing that, Plan B would have the therapist coming to our house to teach Roberto how to use the tool. Again, Roberto would never see the therapist ever again, once he mastered the task. I was ready to follow Roberto's lead. For now, masturbation training is on hold. There have been no concerns in this area since my appointment with the behaviour therapist. Time will tell.

When Domenico left secondary school, he attended two day programs. He brought some of his behaviours with him. One behaviour in particular demanded my immediate intervention. It involved the method of transportation to his day programs. As a student, Domenico rode the school bus for students with disabilities and managed well. The bus driver was the same, every day. The bus was the same, every day. The route was the same, every day. The drive to school was nine kilometres with no traffic lights and few intersections.

Transportation to day programming was arranged through a local company (the only ride in town). Seniors and people with a disability who are unable to drive themselves are eligible for this service. A wheelchair accessible bus, passenger van, or car would be dispatched once a request for a ride was made. Some of the passenger vans and cars are owned and operated by volunteers.

Program G was 14.7 kilometres from home while Program H was 33.4 kilometres. When riding in the wheelchair accessible bus, Domenico's repetitive behaviour of rocking in his seat became more intense. The closer he drew to the day program, the more excited he became. Domenico would rock with greater frequency and energy in anticipation of his arrival. Over time, he added a new behaviour. At every intersection, he would first rock in his seat. He would then tap the window with his index finger and slide his hand down the length of the window. One day, he rocked with all his strength and damaged the seat.

I promised the transportation company that I would do something. I reassured the manager that I would implement strategies the next day before consulting with a behaviour therapist. These strategies included a social story, a picture of Domenico sitting quietly in his seat, a timer to hold his attention, and verbal reminders of the expectations before entering the bus. Domenico understood what was being asked of him but the root cause of the behaviour was locked into his memory. The success was negligible. The behaviour continued. One thoughtful bus driver gave Domenico some fidget items to redirect his focus. This was effective at times, but only with her. The wheelchair accessible bus proved to be an overwhelming experience for Domenico. Every trip was different. Drivers, ridership, and routes changed on a daily basis. The noise (voices, wind, radio, brakes, internal heating and cooling units) and the movement (driving styles, sharp turns, sudden stops, quick accelerations, hills, uneven pavement) presented sensory input that Domenico could not organize or make sense of. Was he rocking to know how much strength was required to receive the same sensory input? Was Domenico's impaired understanding of his body's position in relation to other items and people on the bus contributing to the behaviour? The smell of the diesel fuel could be pushing Domenico's sensory system into overdrive. But for him, it was all in good fun. Domenico was having a ball, similar to riding a roller coaster. In rocking, he may have been asking the driver to go faster or stop harder. Regardless of the cause, the behaviour had to be addressed.

I needed a third voice. I asked for help from a local organization that helps people with disabilities to successfully integrate into their communities. Both the manager of this organization and the manager of the transportation company rode with Domenico on different days in order to observe his behaviour. I also accompanied Domenico on the bus one morning to his day program. The findings from all three of us were consistent with the rocking and tapping that occurred at every intersection. Without someone to encourage him to sit quietly, this behaviour could escalate at any time and without warning.

Together, we came up with a plan. Transportation to Program G was easy. The Passenger Assistant Program (PAP) of the transportation company provides a higher level of support for riders. An assistant rides the bus in order to supervise and aid passengers. As needed, the assistant could verbally remind Domenico to sit nicely in his seat and give him high fives or props when he is successful. Unfortunately the PAP was only an option for Program G because of its location. Program H was out of the PAP's geographical boundaries. Transportation to Program H was therefore limited to volunteer drivers. Volunteer drivers transport fewer passengers and in their own personal vehicle for the most part. A smaller vehicle with less people and minimal stops was thought to be a viable solution. But the behaviour continued. I sent different visual distractions every day. These included photographs and social stories from years past. Domenico leafed through the pictures with interest while en route to Program H, but once finished, the behaviour started up again. Under favourable road conditions, it was a thirty-five minute drive. Under the direction of Domenico's doctor, I replaced one medication for another that has a sedative effect. No improvement. Domenico was trapped in this behaviour of rocking in his seat. Autism had imprisoned him in his own mind. I could see the shackles. Domenico could not help himself. I did not know how to help him. I made an appointment.

The behaviour therapist suggested noise-cancelling headphones. Domenico could listen to music while travelling to and from his day program. This would provide a "bubble" effect around Domenico. The thought behind this suggestion supported the understanding that some people with an ASD have sensory processing deficits. Therefore, eliminating the noise would help him remain relaxed and calm. I purchased a refurbished iPod. Domenico responded positively. He learned how to put the headphones on independently, advance from track to track, and adjust the volume. The rocking however continued at every intersection. There are fifty intersections from our house to Program H along the route I take. I know this because I counted. We have the right of way for twenty-eight. Two have a stop sign and twenty have traffic lights. The behaviour was present at intersections with traffic lights only. I started driving Domenico in the mornings so I could make observations, and I began to see his rocking behaviour as an attempt to interact and communicate with the driver. I asked if the drivers would consider giving Domenico a high five or props at the intersections with traffic lights. This interaction could replace the rocking. We gave it a try. At intersections Domenico still tapped the window and ran his hand down the length of the window, but then he would exchange props or high fives with the driver. It was a lot to ask, I know, but it minimized the intensity and frequency of the rocking behaviour. Domenico was trying to tell the driver that the traffic light had changed. He wanted to "talk" about how much he liked the stopping and starting. Rocking was his attempt at a social communication exchange. Instead of trying to eliminate the behaviour, we found a way to mold it into something more socially acceptable. The intervention strategy was not perfect, but it was a step in the right direction. If only Domenico could stop himself from rocking or tell us how to help him. If only the powers that be would allocate more money to the Passenger Assistant Program to expand its boundaries.

Identifying the reason behind the behaviour is fundamental in developing an effective approach to changing it. In the above example, the source was communicative, sensory, and the innocent amusement of a child trapped in a man's body. The behaviour therapist was part of the solution. I had to bring in other supports and follow through with suggestions made. A collaborative effort made the difference.

*Occupational Therapy.* Occupational therapists help people maximize their participation in everyday tasks such as self-care routines, leisure activities, school, work and all other life roles. Their knowledge of sensory challenges in all daily activities can reduce the negative impact of sensory input through environmental accommodations. People with autism can be under-reactive or over-reactive to stimuli (sight, sound, smell, touch, taste, balance, body in space).

An occupational therapist became involved relatively early in Domenico's and Roberto's lives. Domenico was four years of age and Roberto was two-and-a-half. Her focus was on helping them process the stimuli from their environment so they could remain calm and alert. I remember the very first time she came to our home, two decades ago. Domenico was jumping on the couch pillows that he had thrown to the ground. She built a mountain with the pillows for Domenico to climb and consequently built trust into their relationship, virtually from the word go. Through play, she was assessing his strengths and needs. It was fun, interactive, and effective.

Initially, she came exclusively to our home to provide direct therapy and consultation. Her recommendations were always based on reason and functionality.

We purchased a mini trampoline and a platform swing. A platform swing looks exactly as it sounds. In essence, it is a wide, flat, wooden base suspended by ropes. The trampoline and swing were used during therapy sessions to help with balance, spatial awareness, and positioning of the body. Spatial awareness is the ability to be aware of oneself in a given space and in relation to other objects, including when those objects move. Proprioception is an awareness of where our limbs are in space. Roberto's development of both spatial awareness and proprioception is delayed. He will stare at a ceiling in our house as if he is scrutinizing every last detail. He will hug a wall to help ground him (Illustrated on page 31). Sleep disturbances are common in autism. Developing healthy sleep habits is difficult for people with autism in part because of spatial awareness. I invite Roberto to lie down on the couch when I have a feeling he cannot settle to sleep in his own bed. Whenever he holds his arm up and waves to himself or rolls over on the couch to touch the floor, I know it is going to be another sleepless night.

We also followed her advice and purchased a glider for each of them. Neither could sit still for any significant length of time. The movement of the glider gave them the sensory input they needed while in a seated position.

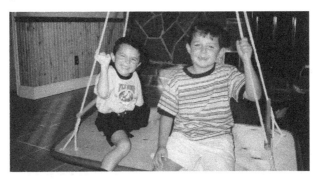

Best of friends, Domenico and Roberto sitting on the platform swing

Soon after the occupational therapist started coming to our home regularly, Domenico began Junior Kindergarten. She turned her attention to Roberto who was home every afternoon. She designed a home program for Roberto, and I hired a support worker to implement the program. This program involved time on the mini trampoline and platform swing, as well as fine motor activities and life skills. One afternoon, she demonstrated how Roberto's vestibular system was under-reactive in comparison to Rocco's, who was two years his junior. The vestibular system is the sensory system involved in coordinating movement with balance. While Roberto was standing, she spun him around several times. He did not stumble or fall to the ground. He was not even dizzy. She then did the same with Rocco. He could not walk a straight line and actually toppled over. This was a normal response.

Roberto's sense of smell was also compromised (and may still be). At a very young age he would approach strangers and smell their clothing. He had to work hard to receive information about his surroundings through that sense. Smelling jars were recommended and introduced. These can be purchased, but I made my own. I picked up some spice containers at a local discount store and put cotton balls at the bottom of each container. I sprayed the cotton balls with my perfume. Roberto found his smelling jars both soothing and comforting. Over time, he no longer sought out the sense of smell in this innocent but socially unacceptable manner. I still use the smelling jars and have since added the scents of coffee and oregano.

Not all recommendations can be sustained. The Wilbarger Protocol (Brushing Therapy) is a program designed to help the person become less sensitive to touch. It has been suggested that this intervention could also help with transitions, attention span, coordination, and self-regulation. A small plastic brush is used over specific areas of the person's body (hands, arms, feet, legs). The process takes three minutes. The face, stomach, and chest are never brushed, as this could result in an adverse reaction such as vomiting. The prescription from the occupational therapist was to brush Domenico and Roberto every ninety minutes. After three weeks, I felt like my arm was going to fall off and I stopped. I could no longer do it (so I had a meltdown moment and then moved on).

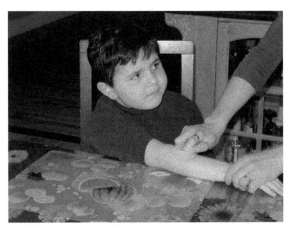

Wilbarger Protocol, I thought my arm was going to fall off.

Once both Domenico and Roberto were at school, the occupational therapist consulted with the school staff. Under her direction, we created a relaxation room within the school. This was a place where Domenico and Roberto could go when they were feeling anxious or simply needed a break. Its doors were open to other students as well. Scheduled visits to the relaxation room were incorporated into Domenico's and Roberto's routines. This reduced the tendency for behaviours to escalate. In the relaxation room, Domenico and Roberto would find calming items such as a glider, a CD player, a mini trampoline, smelling jars, and social stories. The use of weighted clothing and blankets also contributed to their success. During times when they were hyperactive or working through sensory overload, they wore their weighted vests for twenty minutes. The deep pressure grounded them.

The occupational therapist also suggested movement breaks during the day that could be functional. These activities included returning books to the library, bringing the attendance to the office, and running other errands. A shift in their programming gradually evolved to include practical, hands-on learning such as recycling, shredding, and photocopying. The benefits were life-changing. Teachers and peers alike began to see Domenico and Roberto as capable and helpful.

Occupational therapy is not a well-known science. It should be. It gives people the skills for life. It gave Domenico and Roberto a chance to integrate into their school community. Occupational therapy was vital to their success. It is no wonder that our occupational therapist still makes house calls.

*Speech Therapy.* The goal of speech therapy in autism is to improve communication in the areas of comprehension, sound production, expression, and social use of language. Some people may benefit from instruction in sign language while others learn to use picture symbols.

Early development of speech and language includes but is not limited to eye contact, pointing, imitation, and word approximations such as da for dad and muh for mom. Domenico and Roberto had extensive delays in these developmental milestones. Over the years, gains have been made. Eye contact for both Domenico and Roberto is excellent. On the rare occasion, Domenico will point in a communicative manner. Their imitation skills are emerging slowly. Sounds resembling words can only be discerned by a trained ear.

For Domenico and Roberto, speech therapy focused on functional communication. The Picture Exchange Communication System (PECS) remains their main source of communication. We talk about PECS and how it is used in Chapter 8. Over their lifetime, I have worked with three different speech therapists. Each has had expertise in certain areas. The first therapist was very knowledgeable in PECS, the second in school programming, and the third in teaching gestures and word approximations.

I received some training in PECS. I was instructed to set up communication temptations to encourage Domenico and Roberto to use PECS to make requests. An example of a communication temptation is putting a preferred item out of reach. In order to receive the item, they would have to communicate that desire using PECS. Early on in their lives, I drove Domenico and Roberto to a PECS summer camp program. They reached a phase of PECS which involved requesting and never advanced beyond that point. Years later, I drove them to direct speech therapy. We worked on sound production and simple gestures. With repetition, both Domenico and Roberto were learning to nod their heads to communicate yes and turn their heads from left to right in a shaking motion to convey the message of no. I needed to constantly model this communicative gesture for them to imitate or they would forget. And travel to appointments became increasingly difficult. It was a one-hour drive to the therapist's office. It never occurred to me to ask someone else to drive them. How could I? That would involve a minimum commitment of three hours a week. What about winter driving and all the associated risks? They would have to travel on one of the busiest stretches of asphalt in the world: highway 401. I would have insisted on paying them to ease my guilt, but I could not afford it. Speech therapy is $160.00 per hour. I had to terminate the sessions and I still carry that guilt with me today. I hope to resume one day, but question if that day will ever come. I will always wonder if their communication skills would have improved, had services been closer.

The list of treatment options in autism is endless, or so it seems. However, a parent's energy level is not. Neither is a parent's time. There is a ceiling to a parent's financial resources. For this parent, deciding on a treatment plan for my children was the hardest decision I have ever had to make in my life. A prognosis could not be made.

Not then, not now. The outcome of any treatment intervention continues to be ambiguous. Over the lifespan of my children, I will revisit my treatment plan as needed and modify accordingly. The journey has been oppressive at times. While autism has taken me to some very dark places, it has never left me there. Autism helped me develop a formula for living with intention. If you want to know more, turn the page.

Lesson learned - Take guilt out of your treatment plan. As parents, we do the best we can until we know better. Our best is everything. Our best will get us through the day. When we know better, we do better. Work hard. Love with all your heart. Take care of yourself in your own way. Keep going.

# Chapter Seven

## THE TRIAD OF AUTISM
Triple the Opportunity or Trio of Trouble?

---

*It had long since come to my attention
that people of accomplishment rarely sat
back and let things happen to them. They
went out and happened to things.*

---

**ELINOR SMITH**

Autism does not sleep. Autism does not rest. Autism does not even know what day it is. Autism just keeps going and going and going. In order for me to keep going and keep living well with two diagnoses of autism, I constantly challenge the autism triad with my own triad: faith, family, and fitness. This is the formula I apply to maintain my presence of mind and sustain hardiness while fostering a better version of myself.

*Faith.* Faith means believing in God, period! I believe that God has a plan for my life: a divine assignment and a set time to complete it. Faith does not mean complacency, recklessness, or irresponsibility. To this day, I regret dropping out of the nursing programs that I attended for a short time. Little did I know then that my greatest education would come from my sons, Domenico and Roberto. Parenting two sons with autism is the job God gave me. I plan on working every single shift, sights set on a promotion...eternal life with God.

*Family.* I have a large extended family but it feels like one everlasting strong hold. We may live in different cities and towns, but we share the same value system: family first. Although they are not directly impacted by autism to the extent that me and my immediate family are, our parents, brothers and sisters, aunts and uncles, nieces and nephews, cousins and friends all want to understand; they all want to help.

Like you, we gather for the good times and especially for the bad times. For the autistic mind, this presents a challenge to their routine. On some days, even the slightest variance to their schedules can be devastating. Our participation at family functions is therefore dependent on the events of the day or the week or even the hour.

Sometimes I need to send my regrets; sometimes my husband does. A one-to-one celebration of a family member's birthday at another time, for example, is the perfect Plan B: quality time with family while maintaining the daily routine for Domenico and Roberto. I must confess that this balance between what I want to do and what I need to do has left me depleted at times. I feel I am not there for my family. The reality is that sometimes we can make choices, and sometimes decisions are made for us. The difference for me is that I get to choose how I respond. For me, the glass is always half full. I will find a way to do the same thing but in a different way.

*Fitness.* I have committed to some form of exercise since my adolescence. Nothing complicated, nothing expensive. My family room transforms into a state-of-the-art gym the minute I press play and the screen gives birth to my personal trainer. The benefits of regular exercise are well-documented and cannot be disputed. For me, it is a lifestyle and for me, it is life-saving. Annual physicals with my general practitioner often translate into an express confirmation of the status quo.

Every May for as long as I can remember, my breathing becomes laboured. Summer break is just around the corner and you know what that means: a significant change in routine. Domenico and Roberto do not like change. Programming for July and August is not as structured as school. I had a pulmonary function test when my children were still in elementary school to learn why I was gasping for air. There was nothing wrong with my respiratory system then, and there is nothing wrong a decade later. I have identified my laboured breathing as anxiety. I know that once Domenico and Roberto adapt to their summer program, normal respiration will return, no worries. This pattern of extreme panic ended once Domenico and Roberto started day programming (Chapter 10). Their day programs operate twelve months a year, no interruption, no change.

Exercise helps me deal with anxiety by helping me remain positive, healthy, and focused. It is that simple. If not for my regular regime of side planks and stomach crunches, the stress would have killed me – true story. If not the nail in the coffin, then at best, my cardiovascular system would have filed for divorce.

As often as possible, in addition to my workout, I go for a 5.5 kilometre walk with Domenico and Roberto. What could be easier than a walk, right? Wrong! Domenico always walks far ahead while Roberto insists on holding my hand (not that I am complaining). I often call out to Domenico to wait for us to catch up. I am careful not to raise my voice, as it may convey anger and upset Roberto. *Everything is okay, Roberto, Mom is not angry*, I smile in reassurance. Roberto will look at my facial expressions for information. Our walks are quality time, excellent exercise, and the cherry on top. You really do need to stop and smell the roses. During our walks, mine is the only spoken word. Every other sound becomes amplified, every scent intensified. I feel an overwhelming sense of serenity in the stillness of the frozen winter landscape. I see my shadow playing hide-and-go-seek with the summer sun. The autumn leaves dance their best performance for my entertainment and the birds' serenade rings out like it is for me and me alone. Staying fit has kept me alive in more ways than one.

Our lives will be peppered with times of ease and times of struggle. Sometimes, it may seem that we overcome one obstacle only to face another. Do not despair. It cannot rain all of the time. The sun has to come out sooner or later. Life has brought many challenges to my doorstep. In all likelihood, it always will. I am not about to give in. I am not about to give up. I will find a way to get through it. I will make it a life well-lived.

Lesson learned - Believe in yourself and defend your core set of values. Learn who you are and what you are prepared to stand up for! Roll up your sleeves and just go for it – if need be, wear a tank top! And drink lots of water.

# Chapter Eight

## TALKING WITH PICTURES

---

*Just because a man is non-verbal, does
not mean he has nothing to say.*

---

**DOMENICO AND ROBERTO SANSALONE**

Our words are transient and difficult for people with autism to
understand and process. Communication using pictures, however,
is non-transient and can be processed at the pace of the receiver. It
can be customized to mirror the cognitive level of the person and
virtually understood by most, if not all.

Domenico and Roberto, like many people with autism, are visual
thinkers. The three main strategies I have implemented to provide
a visual world for Domenico and Roberto are the Visual Schedule,
the Picture Exchange Communication System (PECS), and the
Social Story.

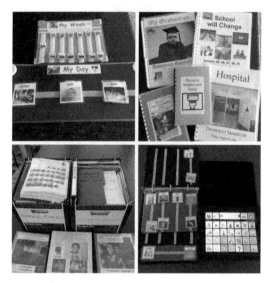

What the non-verbal world of autism looks like

*Visual Schedule.* A daily visual schedule is a critical component in providing structure to the lives of people with autism. This is my voice. This is how I communicate to Domenico and Roberto what they will be doing each and every day and in what order. Picture representations are organized in a linear, sequential manner, from left to right. The visual schedule is tailored to complement the abilities and learning style of the person.

Domenico's visual schedule incorporates the concept of time, modelled after the Time Timer. Roberto's visual schedule is more interactive. A typical school morning for Roberto would read, "Breakfast. Get dressed. Bus." He removes each Velcro picture symbol from his visual schedule one by one as each activity occurs and matches it to the corresponding picture symbol located throughout the house. For example, the corresponding picture symbol for breakfast is at his place setting at the kitchen table. Once the activity is completed, Roberto puts the picture symbol in a finished pouch located just below his visual schedule. "No hard feelings," Roberto reassures his weekend support worker at drop off time as her picture joins the others from the day. "I am finished with you."

To a certain extent, I am a living, breathing, visual schedule for Domenico and Roberto. Domenico follows me around the house, all day long, even to the washroom at which time I ask for space. I feel popular but wonder, *what is a girl supposed to do to get some privacy around here?*

Domenico and Roberto look to me for information, including the events and timelines of their day. I will return home from an outing in haste and immediately change back into my clothes from that morning before "pumpkin time". Like the story of Cinderella, where the transformed coach reverts back to a pumpkin at midnight, "pumpkin time" for me is when I revert back to my role as primary caregiver as Domenico and Roberto return home from their respective programs. The difference between these stories is that mine is not a fairy tale: my story is real. If they see me dressed in formal attire, they become afraid and confused: "Where does she think she is going?" They need to know. When I am dressed in the same clothing from the morning, they know that their evening will follow a predictable routine.

The visual schedule has become an integral part of their success. Their visual schedules even join us on our annual family vacation to Florida. We never leave home without them.

*Picture Exchange Communication System (PECS).* PECS is an augmentative communication system that uses picture representations of preferred items to make requests. This is Domenico's and Roberto's voice. It is their main communication tool. There is variation within PECS. The size of the picture symbol squares can be as small as one inch or as large as three inches. They can be actual photographs, three dimensional objects, or generic pictures. There are phases to move through this system.

Domenico in particular adapted extremely well to the many different formats I created. Under the direction of a Speech and Language Pathologist, I prepared a large board, approximately two feet by two feet, with one-inch picture symbols organized into different categories such as foods, places, toys, and feelings. One day, in his frustration to communicate his needs, Domenico dropped his board on the floor in front of me and pointed with his foot. He wanted his bottle of milk. Now that is what I call talent.

Today, Domenico utilizes his iPad for PECS. Roberto's PECS is organized in a binder format. They have a voice. They have a method to communicate and I am listening.

*Social Stories.* A social story is a book that incorporates pictures to convey a message with minimal script. It is used to teach a skill, change a behaviour, or address virtually any subject matter. Like PECS, there is variation in how the book is formatted.

I have always created my own social stories by utilizing photographs. The very first social story I prepared was for Domenico's first ride on the school bus to Junior Kindergarten. I purchased a small photo album at a variety store. With my Polaroid camera, I took several photographs. I then wrote the story directly on the white strip of each of the Polaroid photographs. It was easy.

When Domenico started grade one, I purchased a laminator and a binding machine. I also invested in a software program called Boardmaker. This computer program has various generic pictures and several applications for those pictures. Later on, I purchased a digital camera. By the time Domenico and Roberto were in grades six and four respectively, I had a library of one hundred social stories.

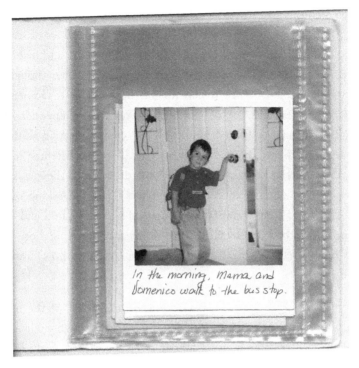

In the morning, Mama and Domenico walk to the bus stop.

First social story, Domenico's first day of junior kindergarten

The merits of a social story were best realized when my third son Rocco wanted no part of toileting. His mind was made up, case closed, until I suggested we make his own picture book. Rocco took a keen interest in the social stories I had prepared to date for his brothers, ranging from riding the bus to going to school and yes, using the washroom. When I asked Rocco if he wanted his own personal and special book about using the washroom, he was more than eager to oblige. He posed for all the photographs, illustrating each step required to use the washroom, and then waited patiently while I put the book together. Once completed, Rocco accepted the condition that he would only be able to read his new book if he agreed to remove his pull-up. Needless to say, he was toilet trained both day and night, no accidents, no turning back, mission accomplished thanks to "talking with pictures."

Implementing these three visual aids into Domenico's and Roberto's lives set me on the pathway to self-awareness. After years of struggling alongside my sons, I began evaluating my ability and inability to communicate. How well did I understand my own thoughts, wants, and needs in order to relay them to others? Unlike Domenico and Roberto whose use of PECS is by rote, I am fluent in the English language. I wanted to improve my communication skills in advocacy of them. They deserved my best. I started listening more carefully to what I was saying with my words, assessed the messages I was conveying, and made improvements. I started asking more questions and sought clarification to ensure I understood and was being understood. I also learned the importance of telling those you love how much they mean to you. The non-verbal world of autism gave me a voice.

The visual world of autism gave me a vision, a view of the life I wanted. Desperately wanting to see the world through their eyes, I considered creating a visual schedule for the events of my day. I looked at my life as objectively as possible. This mental exercise exposed a growing apathy. Day after cookie cutter day, the tasks were the same. The threat of indifference was real. So I focused my attention on the bigger picture of my life, not the here and now. Pursuing new opportunities and interests would have to wait. My responsibilities to my husband and our four children come first and remain absolute. Their happiness and well-being are essential to my own. With love and patience, my turn will come. I know this is true. With this discernment, the monotony of my life faded and my resolve strengthened. Nothing remotely wondrous in the world could take my breath away like the image of my husband and children. The family portrait is my big picture.

Domenico's and Roberto's visual schedules fall short in structuring every aspect of their lives. There is a ceiling to the level that their communication skills will develop. PECS has limits. The applications for using social stories are numbered. Not everything can be represented pictorially.

We, however, communicate in countless ways, including our words. We should use them well. Open dialogue bridges the gap between the pervasive and the known in order to avoid misunderstandings. We also possess the cognitive ability to find the bigger picture of our lives. What is your vision of a life well-lived? Can you develop a visual schedule for your life that will keep you steadfast in the direction of your choosing?

As you endeavour to better understand yourself and those around you, try to be gentle. Empathy is a building block to constructive communication. Everybody struggles, be it internal pressures or external forces, at one time or another. Always reflect back on what you are truly working towards in your life. Add some colour, make a few changes, walk in the light of your own self-discovery, keep the conversation going, and do not simply exist. Live.

Lesson learned - Focus on the big picture – your life – and work on making it a masterpiece. Advocate for yourself, learn who you are, communicate your needs and wants, listen when spoken to, insist on being heard, and keep talking. You have a voice – use it well!

# Chapter Nine

## AUTISM AWARENESS AND THE INCLUSIVE SOCIETY

---

*The true measure of any society can be found in how it treats its most vulnerable members.*

---

**MAHATMA GHANDI**

Confession: I was sitting poolside with another parent. We were watching our children with their respective swimming instructors. Her daughter had autism as well. While exchanging common grievances amongst parents of a child with autism, it happened. I heard her child's noises and they bothered me. The noises of a child with autism bothered me?

*Shame on you, Mirian. Forgive me Father; I know You heard that.*

I wanted to kick myself to the curb for the morning collection. Her child sounded exactly like mine, exactly like Domenico and Roberto. If I practiced intolerance, how could I expect otherwise from strangers who do not live with autism?

The behaviours and vocalization of people with autism draw attention and stares from the general population. Educating others about autism will gradually replace the stares with understanding.

I remember one Sunday in September when Domenico, Roberto, and I headed out to a big-box store to purchase a few household items. This type of environment presents a high degree of stimulation. A visit to this store could potentially result in sensory overload. Our list of things to purchase was therefore condensed to four. We packed our patience and donned our riot gear to brave the crowds. As we made our way through the aisles, single file, I noticed a young boy staring at us. He was staring at Domenico who was making noises. The young boy looked once, and I pretended not to notice. He looked again, and I offered a smile. When he looked a third time, I spoke: "My son has autism. He does not talk. That is why he is making those noises." The boy smiled and looked away.

The outcome of this brief encounter could have been very different. I could have been confrontational and defensive. That would have been the most natural and automatic response. Instead, I walked out of my heart for a moment and into my brain, where I put on the young boy's shoes. This mental exercise helped me understand how natural and automatic the boy's response was to Domenico's noises.

The unknown often manifests as fear. Enlightening others about autism will result in acceptance and inclusion in the long term. Domenico and Roberto attended an elementary school that did not have a contained classroom for students with disabilities. They were integrated into the mainstream student population until secondary school.

Other students would have remained ignorant about autism if Domenico and Roberto had been placed in a contained classroom. I felt that segregating students with autism from the general student population would deliver the wrong message, that they do not belong.

The hardest decisions I have had to make on behalf of my sons involved their programming: mainstream versus segregation, and social communication versus behaviour modification. I opted for the former in both cases and have never questioned my decisions. I believe I made the right choices, but right or wrong, they were mine to make. My sons have to live their lives within the decisions I make on their behalf. Do I feel overwhelmed? You might say that!

So what is my role? How do I ensure my sons become and remain visible and contributing members of their society? An educator once encouraged me to continue advocating for my sons before she assumed a new position elsewhere. I chalked it up to good counsel but was left wondering what form this advocacy should take. Did it mean baring my teeth at the first sign of conflict? Thanks to my incredibly adept dentist, this would be a pleasure, but that is not the way.

Over time, I have learned that autism awareness is a good place to start in promoting inclusion. Within the family unit, at school, and in the community, I have had to be my sons' voice. Though I did not apply for the position, I have inherently understood that it is my job, my divine assignment. I had to educate myself in order to educate others. Two decades later, I am still learning.

A team approach to supporting a student with a disability, in which the parent is an active member, made perfect sense to me. Of course my participation was needed, especially because Domenico and Roberto are non-verbal. But working as a united team did not come easily. I never put the onus on educators to *fix* my children. I never expected the school team to have all the answers and do all the work. There were growing pains that I wanted to be a part of. There was a learning curve for all of us. A shared responsibility between home and school was fundamental to Domenico's and Roberto's success. Having two children with a disability did not give me carte blanch to be disrespectful, unreasonable, or demanding toward anybody. Not then, not now, not ever. Domenico and Roberto were not the only students with a disability. I have a great appreciation for the rights of other students and their families as well as the many responsibilities placed on educators. The day I turn a deaf ear to the cries of others is the day I want to die.

The greatest challenge in the early years of their schooling was in the development and implementation of a modified program. Domenico and Roberto were each placed in classrooms with children their own age, never together until secondary school. While other students were learning multiplication, Domenico and Roberto were counting, matching, and learning about patterns. They were studying the same subject, in this example, mathematics, but academically, they were incapable of completing the same work. Integrating Domenico and Roberto into the classroom was therefore not straightforward. A customized program for each of them required an understanding of their strengths and needs. In order to acquire a working knowledge and profile of Domenico and Roberto, a forum for information sharing was critical. I requested monthly meetings with the school team. They said yes, without hesitation. I started distributing "Minutes of the Meeting" to all members of the team: administrators, teachers, education resource workers, itinerant resource teachers, child and youth workers, special education resource teachers – it takes a village. I would take notes during our monthly meetings, go home, and prepare a written summation of what was discussed, including the next steps. I would follow up regarding the implementation of these steps.

Every September, I would prepare a memo describing their summer programming and would bring the school team up-to-date. I would share any changes to Domenico's and Roberto's overall health. They would be made aware of any new behaviours. The school team came to see me as an involved, hardworking parent and a team player. As we got to know each other better, we discovered that we all wanted the same thing. We all wanted Domenico and Roberto to be integrated into their school community and develop skills for life. We were now on the same page.

From developing a very effective and user-friendly school-to-home communication system, to preparing visual schedules and completing social stories, to providing resources and obtaining input in the areas of speech and language pathology, occupational therapy, and behaviour therapy, I began to evolve as my sons' advocate (having a big mouth helped).

For nineteen years, I sent a daily communication system that I created in a binder format to Domenico's and Roberto's respective programs. There was one page for me to complete, and one for the school. I shared information regarding our evening or weekend, especially noting any changes to the routine. I provided a heads-up if either had not enjoyed a good night's sleep or was not feeling well. Any and all relevant details were conveyed through this system. The school returned the favour and provided me with a window into their day. For me, this daily exchange was second only to the Bible: it was my voice in advocacy of my sons.

One March morning when Roberto was six years old, he accidentally dropped his backpack into our backyard pond. I cared little for his lunch, for it could be replaced. The school-to-home communication system however – my voice – was facing a bone-chilling death. Canadian winters extend far into March. The unassuming pond stood covered with a thin layer of ice. Guess what I did? I frantically removed my boots and jumped in, feet first. I rescued my beloved communication binder from the perils of the Sansalone Harbour just as the bus was pulling up to our driveway. When the bus driver questioned if I had just taken a shower, I replied, *in my parka?* If you are thinking, "She must have been crazy to jump into that frigid water," you are right. I still am a little nuts!

The support and genuine care afforded to me and my sons by the elementary school team were both overwhelming and inspirational. They genuinely wanted to create a program for my sons that would promote their development. They were committed to helping Domenico and Roberto realize their full potential. We had achieved a level of synergy and the sky was the limit: success was enjoyed by all.

Secondary school was a different kind of wonderful. Domenico's and Roberto's placement was in the Planning for Independence Program (PIP). It was seven years in length and organized into four subjects: two subjects were integrated into the general student population and two were contained to the PIP classroom. The building was bigger, the faces were changed, the program differed from elementary school, but my role was the same. The sincere interest and commitment of the school team was very present. Daily communication was exchanged. Collaboration between home and school was upheld. This formula to supporting Domenico and Roberto throughout their lifetime - to be continued!

The reality is that administrators will come and go, teachers will retire, itinerant resource teachers will follow opportunities, child and youth workers will relocate, and education resource workers will be reassigned. They have lives outside of their noble profession of education that will take them out of ours. The dynamics of the team will change, but the method of working together has been developed. Empathy and respect are key. Parental participation is imperative. Daily communication is fundamental. If a communication system similar to the one I created is not possible, try Plan B: e-mail. Today, my daily communication with Domenico's and Roberto's day programs takes place through e-mail.

After secondary school, adult day programming is the next placement for people with disabilities like my sons. Domenico graduated two years prior to Roberto. I met with the respective teams of each of the two day programs that Domenico would be attending. At that meeting, I brought an introductory package which I had prepared for each team member. It included a profile of how autism has manifested in Domenico. I wanted the new team to know that although Domenico has autism, it does not define him. He may be non-verbal, but he has a voice. I prepared a visual schedule for each of the day programs to communicate to Domenico what he would be doing each day. At one program, it follows the First → Then → Last model; at the other program, the visual schedule presents a week at a glance with picture symbols for each hour. I know it is a lot of work, I know it takes time, but then, he is my son.

Domenico graduated secondary school in June of 2013 after a very successful seventeen-year career within the same school board. A student with exceptionalities can remain in school until twenty-one years of age given he or she meets the criteria. Domenico's graduation did not commemorate reaching one milestone and welcoming the next as we know it. He cannot apply to any post-secondary education program. He cannot consider employment, ever. All he can do is look to the adult day programs that are in our catchment area and residential placement down the road, *way* down the road if I have anything to say about it.

Transitioning to adult day programming presented one of Domenico's most significant life changes and thus one of mine as well. I must confess that the thought of taking this step quite literally scared me to death. I was terrified. I was afraid of the unknown and of the person I could potentially become. If I could not secure a smooth transition to my preferred day programs, would I become angry, bitter, withdrawn, depressed? This possibility kept me up at night. I turned my fear into resolve, rolled up my sleeves, and got to work. What choice did I have? We had to move on.

I visited several adult day programs, eight to be exact. I started in the fall of 2012, and by November I had exhausted my list of eligible adult day programs. Only seven months until Domenico's graduation and I was losing hope and struggling to stay positive. In the quiet solitude of my own mind, I prepared Domenico for the uncertainty of what was to come. *Domenico, I went to eight adult day programs. For Programs A and B, you were just a dollar sign. When I walked into Program C, I wanted to walk out immediately. When I walked into Program D, I wanted to run out. Program E was a dream, the Cadillac of adult day programming, but we cannot afford it, Domenico. I would live in a shoe for you, Domenico, but this is completely out of our reach. Program F impressed me, but it is only offered three days a week and not year-round. Program G was a green light, full throttle, but it is only offered two-and-a-half days a week. Program H felt like home, but it has a waiting list. This is a process, Domenico. It may take some time, but we will get there. We just have to hang on and keep going. I cannot change the reality of adult day programming, Domenico, but this I can do: I can work hard, every day, two hands, full heart, big dreams. I promise you that I will not rest. I assure you that I will not stop until I find the right post-secondary placement for you. We will take these next steps together, Domenico, we will find our way.*

When I received the call that Domenico was accepted into the program of *my* choice, I was, of all places, at the salon. The director of the program offered to call me back at a more convenient time but I reasoned that *I will go bald if I have to.* Next to my wedding day and the days each of my four children were born, June 4, 2013 was the happiest day of my life. Today, Domenico enjoys a full week of year-round programming with my top two choices: Programs G and H.

Before I could catch my breath, it was Roberto's turn. He was to graduate from secondary school in June of 2015. Two years had already passed since Domenico had graduated. A new day program was opening in April, and so I attended the January Open House of Program I with Roberto. I was encouraged by what I saw. I was inspired by what I heard. We submitted our application and waited, fingers crossed. Roberto's name was already on the waiting list to join his brother at Program H, fingers and toes crossed. In February of 2015, Roberto had been accepted into both day programs. A full week of year-round programming would be shared between the two. There was still plenty of work for me to do. Great consideration had to be taken to secure a seamless transition. I knew that Roberto would be overwhelmed with all the changes associated with the concurrent start of both programs. Adjusting to one day program at a time would usher Roberto gently into a *true* transition. The support from both day programs throughout the entire process sustained me. They gave me resolution and hope. I pulled Roberto out of school for the final three weeks in June. Instead, Roberto would start Program H in June and Program I in July. I asked Program H if Roberto could visit for one hour, once a week, starting in April. Their doors and their minds opened wide to the idea. I asked the school team if this strategy could be incorporated into his school program, and they answered an unequivocal yes! They would make it work. As a student with a disability in his final semester, the next step of day programming was being introduced gradually. Roberto's transition plan was based on my experience with Domenico. I learned well. I had learned the hard way, but it was better this time. It was different this time. I was afraid, but not terrified. I had a vision of what an effective transition should look like. This time, I asked the right questions. I knew this change was coming. For the past two years I had planned for success. Operation Inclusion accomplished, *for now*. With faith, perseverance, patience, time, and hard work, I faced my fears!

Inclusion into societal programs and services takes money. Participation in a day program carries a substantial fee. Passengers will be charged when transported to and from services. Living in a group home is not free. Parents of a child with a disability are susceptible to personal bankruptcy. Government funding is a subject matter that always seems to hit a raw nerve with the general population. I understand your pain because I feel it too. There is never enough money to go around. The diverse needs of people are endless. But I refuse to jump on that decrepit bandwagon headed toward the dead-end street of despair. This is a coping strategy I have worked on over the years to remain optimistic. I focus on the current good in our lives with gratitude while working towards a better tomorrow. There is government funding for people with disabilities who live in Ontario. As children, Domenico and Roberto both received funding to ensure their participation in community programs. Every year, I had to complete a seven page application, one for Domenico and one for Roberto. If my applications were approved, an amount was allocated. They were approved, year after year. I used these monies to enrol Domenico and Roberto in summer camp. I also hired a Saturday support worker for each of them. This one-to-one support made community involvement possible while providing respite for me. However, the funding did not cover all of the expenses relating to Domenico's and Roberto's disability. The balance was paid out of pocket.

In June of 2013, Domenico aged out of the school system. He was twenty-one years old. The next stage in his life was day programming. He needed money to attend the day programs and money to pay for transportation to each. A lengthy process was required to increase Domenico's government funding to reflect his adult needs. We started in January of 2013 with two interviews at our home. Domenico had to be present. Someone else, other than me, had to be present. Rocco and Jennifer, still in secondary school, were at both meetings in support of their brother. They had to answer questions during the interviews. In July of 2013, Domenico's application was approved and his funding was increased. As far as I know, this government funding will be renewed, year after year, for his lifetime. Should Domenico's needs change down the road, we can apply for an increase.

Roberto, now an adult, has been waiting since February of 2015 for his government funding to increase. His application joined a long list of people needing financial assistance. The list is called a registry. When the government releases funds, an agency looks at the registry to determine who is in greatest need. So we wait and wait and wait for Canada Post to deliver the good news that Roberto's request for a funding increase has been granted. Until that blessed day, we have been selling our assets to pay for Roberto's day programming and transportation costs. The threat to our livelihood is real. But we'll do whatever it takes to support Roberto, even if it means selling our house.

There is much work ahead in promoting autism awareness and developing accessible programming for an inclusive society. We do not live in isolation. We are all connected on some level. Let us be more involved in our own lives and in the lives of others. This participation can begin at home, in our own families. Let us learn to live together in harmony and build partnerships. Let us support each other's wants and needs so that all our lives can be enriched.

Lesson learned - You have a voice and a right to be a visible and contributing member of your world. Participate, keep going, and focus on the forward direction, not the rate of travel. You will get there, all in God's time!

# Chapter Ten

## THERE IS NO PLACE LIKE OUR SECOND HOME
### Day Programming

---

*Home is not a place…it's a feeling.*

---

**UNKNOWN**

For nineteen years, Domenico's and Roberto's classroom was their second home, and mine. School was a place where we felt safe, respected, and heard. For me, faculty members were more than teachers who delivered a curriculum. They were friends who carried a dream. Would I ever find a place like school after graduation? I had no idea what life would be like once school ended. When Domenico entered secondary school, his teachers hosted an information session for parents. A panel of speakers presented options for graduating students. Domenico was in year one of seven. I thought it was premature of me to attend the meeting. But when I received an invitation, I decided to go.

While one speaker addressed the group, another distributed some literature. The first speaker's message was one of caution. There would be no nine-to-five, Monday-to-Friday week, he assured us.

Post-secondary life was very different. The second speaker's message was one of preparedness. As she made references to the literature, she explained that it was never too early to start planning. Seven years would pass quickly, she warned. Included in the literature was a chart outlining a course of action when considering options for post-secondary life. The chart also provided guidelines and timeframes as to when one should visit potential placements and submit applications. Year seven was the time to secure placement or at least get on a waiting list. Placement could be post-secondary education, work opportunities, day programming, or a combination of choices dependent on the person's abilities and interests. The third speaker's message was one of continuing education. A community college program offered additional supports to students with disabilities. There was a prerequisite that students have the ability to successfully complete the course material. Domenico was automatically disqualified from that option. He could not do the work. At this point in the evening, my attitude shifted from hope to fear. Speaker after speaker, the message to parents was the same. Post-secondary life was the responsibility of the family.

This is my message to parents: do not be afraid; just get busy. Get involved. Stay involved. Your constant contribution to your child's happiness and success is the difference. The best advice I received when considering suitable day programs for Domenico and Roberto was to visit the day programs myself, in person. I could see firsthand what the program looks like. I could form an unbiased first impression and ask questions relevant to us.

Day programming offers recreational opportunities as well as life skill development and community involvement in partnership with parents. Both Domenico and Roberto attend Program H, four out of five days a week. Domenico attends Program G one day a week and Roberto attends Program I one day a week. This gives them time together and time apart. The vision and mandate of all three programs uphold the inherent dignity and rights of people with dis-abilities to be active and visible in their communities. In theory, this sounds good. It actually sounds too good to be true, am I right? In practice, it is even better than good: it's great.

Domenico started day programming two years before Roberto. We visited Program H two weeks prior to his start date to trial the new mode of transportation. One staff member approached Domenico upon our arrival. With sign language and a sincere smile, she said, "friend". He does not understand sign language but he understands kindness. A connection was immediately established. Domenico's fondness for this caring woman has grown into a deep friendship over time. He seeks her out of the group and always wants to spend time with her. A picture of them together sits on Domenico's night table. Domenico's transition to day programming was seamless. Together, we worked through some minor issues such as using all his strength when throwing a ball and using too much bathroom tissue.

Roberto's transition to Program H was also fluid, though not without a few ripples. No waves. On his first day, he joined the group for a leisure swim and had a toileting accident. The pool had to be drained. I was devastated. On another day, during a trip, he wandered away from the group. This caused sixty seconds of sheer panic for staff. When I learned that Roberto had ripped someone's clothing, I thought to myself: *three strikes and you're out*. But when I apologized, this is what the program director said to me: "We will continue to work together as we always have in the past to deal with whatever sit-uation arises." I was reassured and resolute but still a little concerned.

On the first day that both Domenico and Roberto attended Program H together, I received a phone call and braced myself for bad news. Much to my delight, the program director had a feel-good story she was eager to share. Roberto, new to the program, was learning the routine. The first order of business upon arrival for all participants is to hang their belongings in the cloak room and then, for those who take medication, to give their pill bottles to the support worker. The support worker then locks all medication in a secure location until it is time to take it. When asked for his pill bottles, Roberto did not respond. Domenico, now a veteran of Program H, took Roberto's pill bottles out of his backpack and gave them to Roberto. Roberto then gave his pill bottles to the support worker with some prompting. Like a caring big brother, Domenico had his back. He wanted Roberto to be successful and had tried to help him. The program director described this tender moment as heartwarming and inspirational. Her enthusiasm mirrored a parent's pride on her child's first day of school. I knew, right then and there, that we were home.

Program H is the brain child of a group of parents with adult children like mine. Post-secondary school options were scarce for their young adults at the time of graduation. Together, they created Program H in 2009. The process was painstaking but the ideology is empowering. Participants of Program H are the salt of the earth, says the founder (I second that emotion). They courageously shoulder a reality so foreign to many, without lament, without resentment. People with disabilities deserve opportunities to live a full life, she maintains. Through advocacy, fundraising, and good old-fashioned hard work, these dedicated parents pioneered a movement of inclusion. They started cautiously with eighteen participants. Six years later, they have reached their capacity and have a growing waiting list. Today, Program H is home to forty participants. There, they come together, as one family, with one common goal: TO LIVE! Look what love can do!

But what happens when there is no love? What happens when the people who run the day programs and group homes have less than noble intentions? Programs C and D left a bad taste in my mouth. I feared for Domenico's and Roberto's safety. I am not saying that I am perfect. I have made mistakes. It has taken me years to forgive myself for being human (and I'm not quite there yet). One evening I became distracted and forgot that Roberto was waiting in the washroom to be bathed. Our routine is that once Roberto finishes using the toilet after dinner, he enters the bathtub, expecting me to appear right away. He had been sitting patiently in the bathtub, naked, waiting for me to bathe him. Fifteen excruciating minutes of sitting and wondering, what could he have been thinking? How easy would it have been for me to just leave him there indefinitely? Who could he tell? He is nonverbal. If someone were to substitute urine for apple juice (his favourite beverage) and then laugh as Roberto started to drink, who could he turn to for help? What if someone were to walk in on Domenico while he is showering or joined him in his bed? What defences does he have? Say it will never happen, please. You know what I am talking about - sexual assault, physical abuse, neglect, abandonment, failure to provide the necessities of life. So many times, these thoughts have kept me up at night. As I listen to Domenico's and Roberto's slumber from the next room, with only drywall separating us, I wonder how I am going to protect them for the rest of their lives. *Rid me of this poison, dear Lord. Tell me no one will ever harm my sons, I am begging you.*

Entrusting my sons to the care of others is a tremendous leap of faith. As parents, we are asked to put our trust in strangers who will care for our very vulnerable adult children. Who do you trust? Trust is earned and trust takes time. The best way to know if you can trust someone is to trust them and be trustworthy.

Some relationships we choose; some relationships are chosen for us. We have family who are more like friends, and friends who are more like family; the bonds we hold dear will continue to change over our lifetime. As we grow through life stages, our inner circle seems to waver in quantity but abound in quality. At least that is what is happening to me. I have entered many social circles in support of Domenico and Roberto. Those who were once distant strangers are now close friends. The greatest investment we will ever make in our lives is time with family and friends. It is not the walls that surround us or the roofs that cover us that define our home. It is only within the chambers of the human heart that we are truly at home. Whatever you call home, be it a person, a place, a dream, or a memory, always remember to reserve a room for God.

Lesson learned - We will encounter many people over the course of our lifetime. Circumstances will thrust us into relationships that would otherwise never come to pass. Some people make it to our future, others do not. They enter our lives for a short period of time either to help us change or for us to help them change. Remember the connections you made, cherish the ones you have, and find your home: there is no place like it.

# Chapter Eleven

## COUNSEL FROM THE CLASSROOM
### So Glad I Asked

*What counts in life is not the mere fact that*
*we have lived. It is what difference we have*
*made to the lives of others that will determine*
*the significance of the life we lead.*

NELSON MANDELA

The Muskoka school trip: one of my favourite conversations with God. Camp Muskoka Outdoor Education Centre is located in Bracebridge, Ontario. During their stay at the centre, students reach curriculum goals while having a blast. The great outdoors is their classroom. I wanted Roberto to join his peers for this three-day, two-night adventure up north. I met with the school team to discuss sleeping habits and possible triggers to behaviour (hunger, fatigue, too much idle time, not enough down time, excessive noise, etc. etc. etc.). Roberto and I made the two-hour drive to take pictures of the campgrounds. I prepared the social story. His bags were packed. It was go time.

As the bus was being loaded, I could not believe my eyes. Amidst all the excitement and commotion, one image immediately brought everything to a standstill. This image virtually brought me to my knees. Two teachers emerged from the school, carrying Roberto's glider.

Both at school and at home, Roberto has a comfort zone – his glider. The rhythmical movement of this type of chair helps Roberto remain calm but alert. With great care and consideration, these teachers secured Roberto's glider into the bus so it would not get damaged in transit. Like devoted parents who would stop at nothing to ensure the family trip was enjoyable to all, these champions gave me great pause. Their thoughtfulness was palpable. I still feel it today!

*Did you see that, God?*

Of course He saw that; what a question! I know God was witness to that display of Christian love. He had hand-picked these teachers to accompany Roberto on his first trip away from his home and family. It was God's idea. Roberto was in good hands; God saw to that!

Parents of students with disabilities are stressed, exhausted, scared, and at times bitter – I get it. But what about teachers of students with disabilities? Ever think they may be working through similar states of emotional unrest?

Any student identified as having an exceptionality, either gifted or challenged, receives an Individual Education Plan or IEP. This is an outline of the student's strengths, needs, supports, and goals. It is reviewed annually. Changes are made in accordance to the student's progress. To be honest, I dreaded the annual IEP review. The severity of my sons' disabilities were discussed out loud and documented. There it was in black and white. No escaping the realities of autism.

Whether in written form or verbally, every time this evaluation was delivered I would cringe at the phrase: "To the best of his ability." Roberto was functioning to the best of his ability: in other words, not doing much. What did I expect? Should teachers tell me what I want to hear, or should they tell me the truth? They should tell me the truth, of course, painful as that may be.

I have expectations for my sons' teachers. I want them to have expectations for me. In fact, I insist educators set the bar high. Give me homework so that I can learn, so that I can change.

Teachers deal with students directly and parents indirectly. They are mandated to deliver a curriculum and they are accountable to administrators. This must be intimidating!

I can only speak to my experience in parenting two students with disabilities. I cannot however speak to the reality of teaching a student with a disability. So I asked.

Stop Crying and Put Your Running Shoes On - Ms. Fearless - One Teacher's Defining Moment

*What has been one of the darkest moments in teaching that caused you to reconsider your career choice?*

I was offered my very first teaching opportunity five years ago. During the interview process, I was asked if I would consider a position in a Planning for Independence classroom. I agreed without hesitation, though I was unfamiliar with the job description. On day one, I thought I was prepared. I thought I was putting my best foot forward by dressing professionally (blouse, skirt, heels). One of the classroom teachers approached me and asked if I owned a pair of running shoes. I wondered why my choice of footwear was in question. She explained that some students attempt to run out of the classroom, and succeed. It took me a minute to process her statement. In my confusion I think I even asked where I was. When she enquired about my understanding of what the Planning for Independence program encompassed, I responded, "Working with students who have learning disabilities?"

She filled in the blanks for me. She described the severity of some of the learning and physical disabilities that we support. She provided an overview of autism (a condition I knew little about), Down syndrome, and other disorders.

When I walked into the classroom for the first time I was immediately grief-stricken. I did not know if I could compartmentalize the inevitable emotional turmoil of the job in addition to the inherent fear.

I was assigned to a student named Matthew. Five years have passed and I can still hear his voice. I often revisit that glorious year together with complete clarity of thought. He was the first student I had ever worked with who had autism. I could not identify any learning or physical disabilities at first sight. He looked like every other student to me. However, it took me only five minutes to realize that Matthew was non-verbal and a runner. He had a heightened sense of touch as well as a fascination for timers.

As the weeks and months passed, a growing endearment for Matthew developed. Despite his tendency to run, which kept me in a constant state of preparedness, he was one of the sweetest students to have ever crossed my path.

One day Matthew had a meltdown. His smiling face became very solemn. He started pacing the classroom. His anger escalated. The Education Resource Workers in the room were encouraging Matthew to sit down, and they were offering him sensory items to redirect his anger. I was horrified. I had never seen this anger before. Matthew then proceeded to bang his head against the wall. I froze on the spot, petrified. Staff responded quickly in an effort to restrain him. When he was away from the wall, he would hit his face with his fist. The workers were successful in bringing him to the couch. He was crying inconsolably. I started crying. This was a first for me. As Matthew sobbed, staff continued to provide sensory tactics to calm him (wet towel on his head, rubbing his temples and hands, deep pressure massage).

Unsure of what to do next, I called the vice-principal for help. She came down to the classroom and asked why I was crying. I gave her an account of the events. She gave me an ultimatum: stop crying or lose my job.

It was in that moment of self-reflection that I questioned my ability to fulfill the requirements of the job. Would I always be the one and only educator to come apart at the seams every time a student had a moment? The vice-principal wanted my decision by the end of the week as to whether or not I would continue working in the Planning for Independence program.

The next day, I asked my colleagues about the frequency at which these types of situations occurred and what caused them. I also wanted to know how they were able to remain emotionally neutral during trying times. I apologized for crying. They laughed in reassurance. Being new to the teaching profession, they explained that I had no experience in crisis intervention or disability. My reaction was therefore normal and reasonable. They maintained that I could do this job.

Matthew returned to class, happy as always. Yesterday was long forgotten (at least for him). It was a new day. Matthew's strength was the answer to the vice-principal's question of my ability to do the job.

I am still teaching in the Planning for Independence program, five years strong. Every day, I make a conscious decision to suppress my feelings, grueling as that is. I focus instead on the well-being of my students, on their feelings. I constantly remind myself that as a proactive and responsible teacher, my job is to provide an environment conducive to learning. When students are in a crisis situation, my first priority is to ensure their safety. I implement all the strategies that I have learned to date to redirect challenging behaviours (sensory tactics, one voice, being firm). I have also learned that this is more than a nine-to-five kind of job. For me, this is a vocation. So yes, I can do this job and do it well.

I wish that vice-principal could see this teacher now. She would see what I see: a hero. But how do they do it? I often wondered how teachers remain committed to their students - assignment after midterm after interview - so I asked. The wisdom that comes with longevity in any aspect of our lives is echoed in the words of this seasoned teacher.

Beyond the Five Senses - Ms. Visionary - A Teacher's Sense of Humanity

*When you think back over your career, was there a moment in time when you felt affirmed as a special education resource teacher?*

Quinn was more teacher than student. He helped me see the human being behind the label of autism. Quinn was highly motivated by the relationship between cause and effect. He always applied his full strength when engaged in sports, climbing stairs, pushing in chairs, and opening doors. Self-regulation was an area of ongoing development. Quinn did not know how physically strong he actually was. He also sought the sensory input this type of behaviour provided. One day, Quinn opened the classroom door with all his force, as per usual. But this time, I was on the other side of that door. Quinn instantly realized that because of his actions, I had come dangerously close to harm's way. Despite being non-verbal, Quinn tried desperately to vocalize his remorse. He hugged me and rested his cheek on my shoulder. I will always remember the sincerity of his apology. He was genuinely sorry. On that day I learned that people with autism are caring and sensitive. They have the capacity for empathy. They feel joy and sadness just like us. They love and laugh, suffer and cry to the same degree we do. A meaningful connection is possible. We simply need to use all of our senses.

*As a fifteen-year veteran, what keeps you coming back to class with a sense of gratitude and enthusiasm?*

I had always wanted to be a teacher. For as long as I can remember, education has been my holy grail. The classroom represents a place of potential and a haven for hope. My interest in special education had unlikely beginnings. A volunteer opportunity placed me amongst students with disabilities. In the months and years that followed, I found myself naturally bonding with my students and their families. Teaching students with a focus on traditional academia rather than teaching students with a focus on functional academia raises the question of quantitative versus qualitative experiences. When academics dominate the curriculum, teachers evaluate test scores and assign grades. With functional learning, teachers, students, and parents all gain an education measured by the development of skills for life. I am privileged to work with these students and their families. No two days are ever the same. The ordinary becomes extraordinary. Our time together is awe-inspiring and life-altering. These students are the most profound teachers I know. These students are truly outstanding.

*If there is anything you could change about educating students with disabilities, what would it be?*

Students with disabilities deserve to have choices for post-secondary opportunities. The four-year secondary school program prepares the general student population for higher education. They are encouraged to exercise their right to access one of the prolific college or university programs available. For students with disabilities, however, their secondary school experience prepares them to live and thrive independently within their communities. The school program should focus on teaching them employable skills, paid or volunteer. Their school experience should explore hobbies for leisure time and develop practices for healthy living. I would like to see more opportunities for students with disabilities outside of the school environment.

When I thanked Ms. Visionary for her insight, I told her that I would like to see more teachers like her.

Education Resource Workers (ERWs) are integral members of the school team. They provide direct assistance to students with disabilities (physical, developmental, behavioural). Many students with a disability follow a modified program with the support of the ERW. This allows the classroom teacher to focus on delivering the standardized curriculum to all the other students. ERWs are role models, mentors, and friends to their students. They are the ones who greet students at the start of each school day. They are the ones who sit side by side with their students all day long. And they are the ones who wish them a good evening at the end of the school day. It is no surprise that attachments are often formed between ERWs and students. Sometimes parents make a connection with an ERW. I did. I developed a strong bond with one extraordinary ERW. I wanted to know if she felt the same connection with me, so I asked.

He Will Be Great - Ms. Faithful - One Educator's Sacred Connection

*How do you see your role as Education Resource Worker?*

> My first placement was in a grade two classroom. That was fourteen years ago. Before that I worked in a day care setting for ten years, though never with a child with a disability. I had no clue what I was getting myself into. The student I was assigned to had non-verbal autism, and a developmental disability as well, but his eyes spoke a million words. It was love at first sight for me (and I think the feeling was mutual). His smile melted my heart. I relied on observations to get to know him. I noticed my student's gaze shift as we sat in the classroom. Every now and then, he would smile at me and I would smile back. It was during the silent spaces between

the smiles that my role became crystal clear. He needed me to be his voice of advocacy. He needed me to translate the foreign language of the non-autistic, verbal world. His ability to integrate into a mainstream classroom was dependent on my ability to build a bridge.

My student was to receive his First Holy Communion that June. We practiced all year long. When the day finally arrived, I was so nervous. But I just knew in my heart that he would be successful. I prayed all the way to the parish. I arrived to complete darkness, but the power outage was thankfully resolved in time for the sacrament to proceed. I reassured his mother that he would be great and he really was. Though he was ordinarily unable to remain focused for more than five minutes at a time, on this evening he smiled his way through an entire two hours of reverence. Though he had a heightened aversion to several food textures, he accepted the host with grace. At the completion of the ceremony, he brought his hand up to his tie in a request to change into more comfortable clothing. My eyes filled with tears. It was one of the proudest moments of my career.

When describing my role as Education Resource Worker, the analogy of a pillar to a bridge holds true. A pillar needs strength in order to support the bridge. Without the pillar, the bridge cannot sustain itself. Without the bridge, the pathway to any place worth going is lost. I have to be there for my students. They deserve my best. I want to give them every opportunity to reach their true potential. I work for them. I do not stop when I am tired. I stop when the work is done.

*How can parents help you in your role as Education Resource Worker?*

Parental involvement is paramount. Ongoing communication is fundamental, especially for students who are non-verbal. Consistency between home and school is critical for the student to progress. If my expectations differ from those at home, the student may be confused. When strategies are shared, the student will have the tools for success. There will be growing pains but there will also be learning and progress. As a united team, the student will thrive.

*What is the most challenging aspect of your role?*

Students with autism struggle with a variety of stimuli, making it difficult for them to remain calm and engaged on a given day. A poor night's sleep, a certain weather system, or a shirt that does not feel right all have the potential to enthrall the student. At these times a connection with my student may be compromised. I feel challenged when confronted with sensory issues that I cannot change or identify. We endure, we adapt, we learn, we make the most of the day, and we move on. We overcome.

This exceptional ERW believes in her exceptional students. She rallies behind them. She gives them a voice. She connects them to their potential. If you met her, I am sure you would agree: SHE IS THE GREATEST! Her first student, fourteen years ago, was Roberto.

Long after graduation from secondary school, when Domenico and Roberto no longer walk the halls of their second home, fond memories carry on. When feeling discouraged, I revisit the moment Roberto's ERW rushed to his side and asserted, "He will be great."

On days when the thief of fatigue threatens to rob me of my resolve, I reflect back to the day Domenico's teacher dropped to her knees and cleaned the cobwebs off an abandoned study carrel. This carrel was to become Domenico's quiet place. Its structure would shield him from visual distractions and keep him focused. If I ever lose my will to go on, images of all the smiling faces from years past will reignite my fire. I will even draw strength from the times we were at odds, for it was during those times of division that we learned how to work as a team.

If I had not asked about the realities of educating student with disabilities, I would have overlooked the daily hardships teachers inevitably encounter. If I had not tried to put myself in their place, I would have concluded that teachers simply put in their time. Had I turned a blind eye to the forever changing dynamics of the classroom, I would still be in the dark. If I had not asked, I would not have known. I am so glad I asked!

Lesson learned - The student is always the core focus of any relationship between home and school. A partnership of shared responsibility, mutual trust, and ongoing respect will best support the student. Within this partnership, there is room for human error and human forgiveness. Together, let us get to work for our students so they can get to work on building a life for themselves.

# Chapter Twelve

## CHANGE IS THE ONLY CONSTANT

*In the waves of change we find our true direction.*

**FELIX HOI**

Routine, routine, routine – for the autistic mind, this is gospel. People with autism resist change, fear change, struggle with change. I think we all do to a certain extent; I know I do. It is the uncertainty inherent in change that translates into anxiety and my need for familiarity. For Domenico and Roberto, change presents a very real threat to their sense of security. They thrive within a predictable routine, but can it be sustained?

From bus delays to cancellations, inclement weather to power outages, staffing shortages to absenteeism, illness to loss, and countless other disruptions, life happens and change is indeed the only constant. Something as logical as layering one's clothing presents a challenge for Domenico and Roberto simply because it represents a change. The autistic mind reasons that, *if I wear my jacket in the morning, I wear my jacket in the afternoon*, even if the temperature difference is significant. Asking Roberto to remove his jacket mid-way through our walk is asking a lot on some days. "Mom likes to live on the edge," Roberto is probably thinking.

How do I help Domenico and Roberto develop the life skill of coping with the inevitability of change? After years of hands-on experience, I came up with an action plan that I follow religiously. I am constantly evaluating and modifying four strategies.

*A predictable routine.* Establishing a predictable routine at home is fundamental to Domenico's and Roberto's overall well-being and success. It affords them the structure they need to feel safe. I have little to no control over what happens when they walk out the front door. However, within the sanctity of our home, I take control. When they return from their respective programs, they have an expectation that I will be there. For Domenico and Roberto, I am the constant. For me, God is the constant. They know that dinner will be served at five. Bath follows dinner, then evening snack, downtime, and finally bedtime. Their visual schedules tell the tale of a typical day. Domenico and Roberto are grounded to a certain degree when offered a predictable routine, something they can count on to remain the same. They have confidence in me that, should their routine differ from normal, I will prepare them. This has helped them develop frustration tolerance for times when they are not prepared. I have earned their trust; consequently, Domenico and Roberto are better able to adapt to a world that continues to threaten them. When they walk through the front door at the end of their day, they know that *Mom is on the job.*

*Subtle changes to the routine.* Incorporating change within a well-established routine is to the autistic mind what antiseptic is to the wound. It may sting initially, but things will not get better if we insulate ourselves from the stress of change. A static world is unrealistic. Once I had cemented a regimented schedule into the foundation of our lives, I started introducing subtle changes. To Domenico and Roberto, these changes were monumental. Developing the ability to accept change as a constant probability, not an enemy, will enhance their quality of life. Change is inescapable, as life adopts a perpetual and progressive momentum. Therefore, when it makes sense to do so, I switch things around. If we turn right at the bottom of our drive-way when we start our walk, we go the distance of 5.5 kilometres. When we turn left, we only walk for 3.3 kilometres. Nine out of ten times, we go the distance. Every now and then, we take the short cut. Most of the time, I brush Domenico's teeth. On days when he seems receptive to the challenge, I encourage some independence. The majority of the minor changes I make involve the location of items in their surroundings known as environmental prompts. On Friday afternoons, Domenico's and Roberto's backpacks go into the closet for the weekend. Rocco's and Jennifer's backpacks go in their bedrooms. On Sunday nights, all four backpacks emerge well-rested and line up in single file for the Monday start. I often rush to put all my groceries away before Domenico and Roberto return home. Sometimes I leave a few bags out so that they can see and understand that "Mom went out today." Domenico and Roberto are able to manage well for the most part because change during their lifetime has come gradually and by design.

Other small modifications are necessary in order to develop a skill such as communication. In place of PECS, on occasion I accept a communicative gesture like pointing. Domenico and Roberto are making the change in a safe environment. They are in control this time. *How affirming.* It may slip my mind (intentionally) to put utensils on the table. This communicative temptation presents an opportunity for Domenico and Roberto to "talk" about what is missing.

Some people with autism attach a behaviour to a routine. Whenever we go to our local pharmacy, Domenico has an expectation that we are picking up medication. He hits the concrete wall of the building with his hand as we make our way to the front door. He likes the feel of the bumpy exterior. One Sunday afternoon, I had to mail a letter. The main post office was closed. Anticipating that using the post office at the pharmacy would confuse Domenico, I parked in a different location than usual. When entering the pharmacy, I deliberately walked down a different aisle, away from the pharmacy counter. The change of visiting the pharmacy for another purpose was seamless. Domenico did not hit the exterior wall because we had parked somewhere else. We had changed the routine.

In an effort to break some of their obsessive-compulsive tendencies, I vary the way we do a familiar activity. When he was younger, Domenico was preoccupied with the laundry basket. He was unable to quiet his mind to sleep at bedtime until I had folded and put the laundry away. I became very silly in order to shift his focus. It was fun being a clown. I would fold the laundry and leave the empty basket in the middle of the hallway. Sometimes I would kick it like a soccer ball because it was in my way, *Mom scored*. I would walk around the basket, in the basket, and over the basket. Other times I left the basket in the bathtub, turned it on its side, and put my groceries in it. I kept him guessing until he finally dismissed me: "Mom has fallen into the abyss; goodbye, Mother." Incorporating minor variations to their normal routine and environment has educated Domenico and Roberto about change. Change is not to be feared but rather anticipated. The task will be accomplished, just in a different way. In life, it is often the accumulation of little things we do that has the greatest impact.

*Visual Preparation.* Whenever possible, visual preparation for any change is essential to Domenico's and Roberto's advancement. A one-page visual will be sufficient in some situations in place of a social story. The use of the universal "no" symbol is very effective in communicating that something is not available. You have probably seen this symbol of a red circle with a diagonal line through it superimposed over a picture to communicate a message such as 'No parking.' I use this symbol extensively to prepare Domenico and Roberto for a change, such as a teacher's absence. I often do not know who the replacement will be. The one-page visual will therefore include a written statement of reassurance such as, "A new friend will help me." Although they may not understand the text in part or at all, the pictures that support the text lend to a more complete explanation for the change.

I prepared a booklet with pictures of community places such as the grocery store, the pharmacy, the shopping mall - all the places we frequent. Like a faithful friend, this booklet stands at the ready and has taken permanent residency in my vehicle. Before heading out, I open the booklet to the appropriate picture and hand it over to Domenico and Roberto. Pictures do not disappear like our words do. They can refer back to the picture while we drive to our destination and start thinking about the associated expectations. "The grocery store is always crowded. Crowds make me uncomfortable. I am going to try to stay calm."

In addition to the visual schedule, I created a weekly schedule and a monthly calendar. These provide Domenico and Roberto with a week at a glance and a month at a glance. Mondays are challenging days for all of us, and Domenico and Roberto are no exception. It seems that on Mondays they need to relearn what is expected of them. The weekly visual schedule prompts them to start preparing mentally. The monthly calendar effectively gives them warning of an upcoming social event, a long weekend, or a holiday. Every morning, they cross off the date on their calendars. When Domenico and Roberto remain in the "know" as much as possible, their anxiety levels about change are reduced.

*Plan B.* In anticipation that plans may change, I develop alternatives. Idle hands governed by the autistic mind are an exercise in despair. With limited abilities and limited interests, how do you pass the time in a positive and functional manner when the schedule is different? When a power outage is probable, I charge their electronics ahead of time so they will have some entertainment. If there is not enough time to go for a walk, we use the treadmill instead. When I know Domenico and Roberto may have to wait to see the doctor, I bring an iPad for Domenico so his favourite animated friends can keep him company. I bring an iPod Shuffle for Roberto so he can enjoy his favourite tunes should the wait be longer than expected. I take the first appointment in the morning or the first appointment after lunch to minimize the wait whenever possible. I schedule all appointments well in advance and at intervals so that I can visually prepare them without overwhelming them. When I think ahead, when I have a back-up, when I develop a Plan B, I am planning for success.

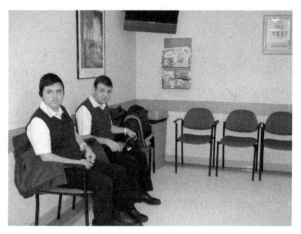

Domenico and Roberto waiting their turn for blood work

Caught between two polar opposites of predictability within the world of autism and diversity within a changing world, I evolved. Autism has effectively and painfully propelled me out of my comfort zone. Quite honestly, I think a life without autism is, well, a little boring! I prefer the creativity and think-outside-the-box approach to living with autism over the potential stagnation and complacency of living without autism. What I could not change ended up changing me. I changed the way I think. The human computer, my brain, is decisively my greatest tool.

I now make a conscious decision to find opportunity in every challenge. I search for the reason why something is happening and welcome a new understanding. It takes practice. It takes discipline. Perhaps you can relate to the unpredictability of inclement weather. Students pray for it; parents just pray. I remember one snow day in particular. Roberto's bus was cancelled, and there was no school. This was a last minute change. I could have chosen to be miserable. That would have been the easiest thing to do. Instead, I saw this as an opportunity for one-to-one quality time with Roberto, as Domenico's transportation to his day program was still a go. Once Domenico was on his way, Roberto and I left for our walk. We owned the road. The side streets had yet to welcome the morning commute. Our footprints followed the road less travelled. Who wants to go for a walk in a snow storm? *Not me.* I questioned whether following God's plan for our lives had actually played out like a snow day. I had my own agenda for that day, but Mother Nature had delivered a snow storm. I had intended to return to school once my children were independent, but God assigned autism to be my education. God's plan, I later learned, is the plan. God's plan, I now know, always prevails. On that snow-covered Wednesday, we turned right: we went the distance.

The world of autism demands we anchor our lives and stay the same. The real world insists we fasten our seatbelts and hang on for dear life. We are in for quite a ride. Autism has helped me differentiate between what I can influence and what is out of my control. I cannot alter the realities of autism, but I can shape how I live with autism. I can change myself. I can learn who I am at my core and build on that understanding. Self-awareness is one of the gifts of living with autism. I have embraced the privilege of choosing what changes I am going to make. What other choices have I made? You ask the best questions, thank you.

Lesson learned - Make it your business to change. Change the way you think; adjust the lens through which you see your life. Our personal perception of our lives is a powerful agent of positive change once we commit to seeing the glass half full. Improve your attitude so that in turn you can alter your behaviour. Celebrate the personal growth that will follow, and start living the life you were intended to live. Love your life.

# Chapter Thirteen

## OUR CHOICES HAVE CONSEQUENCES

*We either make ourselves miserable, or we make ourselves happy. The amount of work is the same.*

**UNKNOWN**

I choose to see the glass half full, but it takes courage. My husband seems to have twenty/twenty vision when it comes to being optimistic (but do not tell him that). As far as that man is concerned, I am Mother Teresa.

Our choices have consequences. I chose to terminate my employment twenty years ago and stay home with my children. It was the right choice for me. It was the easiest decision I have ever made, but it came at a price, and I am still paying. In life, sometimes the right choices and the hard choices are the same. Let me explain. I knew that the severity of my sons' diagnoses necessitated all of my resources. It was clear to me that they needed me to be home with them full-time. I also realized my need to be their primary caregiver. I remember when I was still working at the hospital and Domenico and Roberto were both attending the daycare located on hospital property. This daycare was for children of hospital employees as well as the community at large. Domenico was in the preschool room and Roberto was in the infant room. Domenico needed one pair of shoes to wear inside the daycare setting and one for outdoor use. I drove to a nearby mall during my lunch hour one day to purchase a new pair of shoes. I gave the childcare worker the shoebox and rushed back to my office. When I picked Domenico up at the end of my work day, I went to change him into his outdoor shoes. As I removed his new shoes, I noticed that the paper packaging was still stuffed in his shoes. Domenico's feet had been squished in the shoes with the paper. He had worn them that way all afternoon. Childcare settings are busy places. Domenico, being non-verbal, could not say anything. I could have (and should have) taken the time to put the new shoes on Domenico myself after purchasing them. But I didn't want to be late for work. Domenico's (and Roberto's) dependency and inability to speak up for himself is a reality that contributed to my decision to stay home. I understand that now. I didn't then. I simply internalized the experience. All I knew when I decided to terminate my employment is that the road ahead would be uncharted and the travels rough. I knew I wanted to be the one who waves good-bye every morning and the one who welcomes them home every afternoon. Knowing my priorities was the easy part of the decision. The hard part came in accepting what I was giving up by staying home: financial gains, skill development, societal participation, and community involvement.

Early into my decision to stay home, I became afraid of losing my individuality and identity within my role as primary caregiver. I felt like an extension of someone else's needs. Though I chose to stay home, as the years passed I longed to find my true purpose. I was drowning in a tidal wave of responsibilities. I have a household to run. I have two other children who need me. My husband needs me. I need time to be me. The perpetual To-Do list insists I focus on the task at hand. When Domenico and Roberto are at their respective programs, I work towards shortening my To-Do list. I go a little crazy. I open doors that Roberto insists must stay closed. I return the towel on the vanity in my washroom. I relocate the towel that hangs at my work station, the kitchen sink. Roberto needs to see it there at all times. I leave papers out so I can go back to them during the day. I turn the radio on so I can listen to my favourite all-news station (I like to be in the know). I call family and friends for a gab session. My voice can be loud (and it is; my mouth is that big). I meet a friend for coffee or invite them over to visit as I cook. I do a workout, go grocery shopping, run other errands, and schedule doctor appointments for myself. On some days, I literally run around the house, trying to get the entire day's work finished before they return home (dinner prepared, table set, change of clothes waiting, evening snack ready, lunches for the next day made). Once they return home, I work for them. I suspend my list in order to maintain a predictable routine, in a somewhat static environment, for their benefit. I make no telephone calls in the evening unless absolutely necessary. I do not run from room to room in the house. I try to stay quiet as much as possible, and when I do talk, I try to maintain a low-pitched voice. And I try to smile big. I try to keep the environment calm and orderly and the mood positive. This is more than a full-time job; this is a calling. In my desire to better understand autism, I started looking at myself as objectively as possible. I discovered that I needed a positive outlet to counterbalance the harsh realities of autism without which I would surely falter.

My heart was playing a game of tug of war with my brain. I wanted to be home whenever all four of my children were home. Domenico was in grade three, Roberto in grade one, Rocco in Senior Kindergarten and Jennifer in Junior Kindergarten. This translated into a very small window of time to do anything for myself. I turned down offers from family members who were willing to care for the children so I could take a university course or join a local gym, two possibilities I tossed around. It was an awesome responsibility, I thought. Introducing another caregiver would confuse Domenico and Roberto especially. And it would have to be taken on as a job without pay, not just a helping hand every now and then. They would have to commit to a regular work schedule, once a week for example. I could not bring myself to ask for that type of commitment from anyone in my family, and I didn't. I did however rely on government funding to hire a support worker for Domenico and a support worker for Roberto. Ten years later, I trust them completely. As needed, I also hire other support workers who have come in and out of Domenico's and Roberto's lives over the years so that I can attend weddings, funerals, milestone birthdays, and the like. I wanted to be home whenever my children were home, end of discussion! (Did I mention that I'm stubborn?) What personal pursuit could I possibly undertake with this self-imposed time constraint?

I waited until Jennifer started full day elementary school to delve into interests outside of my parental responsibilities. As I moved from task to task each day, I considered my options. Would furthering my education be fulfilling? Could I pursue a university career and still care for my family? Would hobbies fill the void? I thought about registering for online courses, but to what end? A four-year university online degree program would take considerable time to complete, and later, after graduation, what would I do with my diploma? I like to exercise, so I registered for ten sessions with a personal trainer. But as Roberto began struggling through some changes of his own, I shelved the idea. I love singing, but I cannot sing, at least not well. Roberto finds music soothing. I wanted to sing to him – not torture him – with my rendition of Led Zeppelin's "Stairway to Heaven", so I started taking singing lessons. Then a family member was hospitalized and faced an extensive recovery. I stopped the lessons.

I have always had an interest in the health care profession. Knowing that the hospital setting remains a place of healing and service for me, I volunteered at a nearby hospital in the fall of 2012. Shortly thereafter, I was offered an employment opportunity. It afforded me the flexibility and comfort of working in my own home and within my own schedule. I accepted the position with some trepidation about my ability to fully commit to both work and family responsibilities. Unfortunately, volunteering and working from home proved to be a recipe for burnout. With reluctance, I hung my volunteer vest in the closet, vowing that one day I would return to work. In September of 2014, Jennifer entered her graduating year of secondary school. Fourteen years had passed. What gains had I made towards achieving my personal ambitions since my youngest child had started grade one? I had exhausted my options, or so I thought. Eventually, I began to seriously consider the suggestion from family, friends, and strangers to share my story about living with autism. I knew that this time, I would go all the way. I made an important decision: this time, I would not quit.

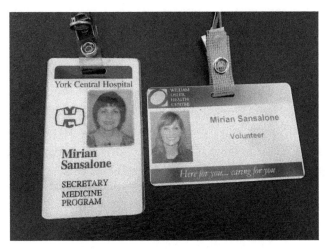

Sixteen years later, Same dream, different hospital

I made choices for my life that I will defend to this day. I will continue to make decisions for my life. Domenico and Roberto, on the other hand, will never develop the cognitive ability to make real choices in their lives. They have to live within the choices I make for them. I feel that I am not qualified to make such monumental decisions for my sons, and I often have more questions than answers. I regress, I succumb, I cry every day - sometimes the gentle ripples of a quiet river, some days a tsunami - but I keep going, never stopping. Sometimes, when the only choice you have is to soldier forward with a brave heart, you begin to realize your true potential. I may never return to a university lecture hall. I doubt I will ever exercise outside of my family room. In all probability, I will never learn to sing. But I do have a bucket list. And I still intend on singing, just not when anyone can hear (that would be cruel). There are ten items on my bucket list. The first is to be God's humble and faithful servant. The last is to take care of Domenico and Roberto for the rest of their lives. My choices are clear.

The ultimate life-changing decision I have made for myself is to develop my character, to remain of good cheer, and to be humble and grateful in any situation. I want to become someone God would be proud to know. Nothing is more empowering than knowing someone is happy because of me. When I give of myself, I often receive so much more in return. My greatest hope is to be remembered as a spirited person who offered her best smile to every single person she encountered in her lifetime, even if she did not feel like it, even if they did not deserve it. Note to self: I owe it to my family and friends to live my best life, I owe it to God, and I owe it to myself. Helping others live their best life defines living my best life, so here I go!

Lesson learned - Take responsibility for the choices you have made, define them, defend them without reservation, and be proud of them. Be proud of yourself. Respect yourself.

# Chapter Fourteen

## MY YOUNGEST CHILDREN

*The giving of love is an education in itself.*

**ELEANOR ROOSEVELT**

They say that growing up is hard to do. What would they say about growing up with two brothers who have autism.

I hear myself say it over and over again: *I have four children. Two have a severe form of autism, and then I have two other children.* Two other children, born into a family of strengths and challenges. They too have strengths and challenges. Everybody does. All too often, however, Rocco's and Jennifer's needs have been shelved, compromised, forgotten, and yet they still love their brothers unconditionally.

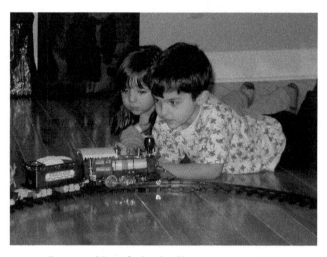

Rocco and Jennifer by the Christmas train, 2001

How might their relationships have matured over time? What kind of men would Domenico and Roberto be today if they were not born with autism? I have tried to picture it. I have closed my eyes, disassociated all other thoughts, and welcomed images of a twenty-five-year-old Domenico driving to work or a twenty-two-year-old Roberto preparing for a night out with friends. I have willed these images to come to life in my mind's eye. They would not make me sad. But as hard as I try, I cannot make it happen to save my soul. When I watch Jennifer in action, however, I cannot help but notice some of Domenico's qualities. They would have been a united force. Every time I sit down for a heart-to-heart with Rocco, I feel it would have been the same between Rocco and Roberto. They would have shared many a laugh together.

Domenico and Roberto enjoy an unspoken comradery because of their similarities. They find comfort in each other's company, and they are well aware of what the other is doing at all times. Roberto behaves as though he is the older brother. When Domenico reaches for a second helping at the dinner table, for example, Roberto will gently move his hand away. Roberto will only tolerate his and Domenico's ball caps on the coat rack, one on top of the other, even though it has four hooks. Nobody else in the family is allowed to leave their belongings on the coat rack. Domenico becomes genuinely concerned whenever he sees his brother struggling. He will go up to Roberto in an effort to read his facial expressions and then turn to me as if to say, "Help him." When asked to set the table, Domenico places napkins, utensils, and glasses for himself and Roberto only. Equally endearing is the bond between Rocco and Jennifer. Sibling rivalry was virtually non-existent as they were growing up, and their adoration for one another still holds true to this day. Rooted in love and respect, there is a sincerity in the connection they hold sacred. Life would have been very different for the four of them if not for autism, but would it have been better?

I remember attending the Geneva Centre for Autism Symposium over a decade ago. I wanted to better educate myself about autism. Geneva Centre for Autism is a global leader in providing services to people with an ASD. They also offer courses and training events for professionals and families. At the symposium, a sibling panel shared personal experiences in living with a brother or sister who has autism. I was all ears, as Rocco and Jennifer were still in elementary school at that time.

A young woman addressed the group with great familiarity and confidence. She spoke of her older brother and how her mother would leave her to *babysit* while she enjoyed some respite and adult interaction. This young woman, a mother herself at that time, resented the responsibility. She finally convinced her mother to put her brother in a group home, asserting that her mother *had done this long enough*. I could not believe what I was hearing.

Who is in a better position than me, their mother, to know when I have had enough? There is no doubt that parents of children with autism are casualties of burnout. The feedback I receive from those who truly care about me matters, and I do listen. With that being said, this is my lifelong job. I do not mind putting in the overtime. I will even take the night shift if necessary, whatever it takes to get the job done. I work for God. He will tell me when to retire.

When I shared the Geneva Centre sibling panel story with Rocco and Jennifer as young adults, they had a lot to say. I would like to introduce you to my two younger children.

*What is the best part about having two brothers with autism?*

> Rocco: Domenico and Roberto have given me an entirely different outlook towards life. I have learned to not be so judgmental of others. Also, they are quite possibly two of the most kind-hearted guys out there; they would never hurt a fly, and that's something that I don't see very often anymore.

> Jennifer: They bring out the best in everyone, even those who you wouldn't expect to have a heart. I love hearing how they've touched the lives of others. They are very able and have taught others so much about autism. I have developed life skills that I would not have learned anywhere else.

*What is the hardest part about having two brothers with autism?*

> Jennifer: The most difficult part is realizing that they were born with autism, and I was not, and I can't do anything about that. Seeing how uncomfortable they are sometimes in their own skin is also very painful. I struggle when the reality and extent of their disability manifests in front of my eyes at unexpected and random times. I find it difficult when I see others being disrespectful towards people with autism or any other disability for that

matter. I don't like hearing their rude jokes and how they laugh and stereotype them.

Rocco: Accepting as absolute that some questions will never be answered is probably the hardest part about having two brothers with autism. What would life have been like if Domenico and Roberto did not have autism? Would it have been better? I'll always wonder. My brothers have shaped who I am as a person and the manner in which I have lived my life to date. For this, I am truly grateful. But the tough times that inherently speak to the realities of autism hurt because reality is something we often do not like to face.

*What have you learned from having two brothers with autism? What impact has it had on your life?*

Rocco: Having two brothers with autism has taught me that everything in life happens for a reason and that we need to make the most of our opportunities in life. If God felt we couldn't handle the hardships that come with the situation we are in, He wouldn't have brought us together as a family. Domenico and Roberto have impacted my life in ways that nobody else has. They have helped me understand that although we have the ability to communicate, we often fail to do so, and they will always try to communicate with us. They've shown me that sometimes in life the 'impossible' is actually very possible.

Jennifer: I have learned to be more patient and not take things for granted, to be grateful for what I have. Domenico and Roberto have had a positive impact in helping me overcome some major setbacks because I see how hard they have to work to accomplish the simplest of tasks. My non-verbal methods of communication have improved and I better understand why actions speak louder than words. They have taught me the value of planning ahead and following a routine. My first tattoo will be the autism ribbon with Domenico's and Roberto's names written beside it.

*If you had the power to change things, would you take autism away from them?*

Jennifer: I love my brothers for who they are, and I would never change them. Autism is a big part of what makes them so amazing. I refuse to picture my life any other way. I would not have my head on my shoulders or be as connected to my family if not for them. I would not be as respected, taken seriously, or integrated into my community if not for them. I have a greater circle of friends because of them. Formal education has not taught me what they have. They give my life purpose. They inspire me to live, not merely exist.

Rocco: No, most certainly not. My brothers have truly had an amazing impact on my life. Of course, there have been rough patches along the way and the likelihood is that there will be more tough times in the future. Despite that, the memories I have of my brothers and the lessons they have taught me are priceless. Their smiles — their ability to put smiles on the faces of others, even perfect strangers — is something I truly treasure. I wouldn't change that for the world.

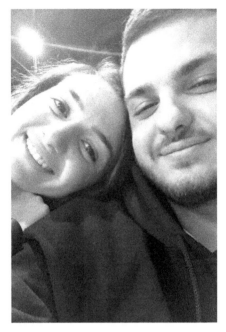

Rocco and Jennifer, Family who are more like friends, 2017

ENOUGH? The speaker at the Geneva Centre sibling panel felt her mother had cared for her brother long ENOUGH! She had insisted that the time was now to place him in a group home. I wish Rocco and Jennifer could have been on that sibling panel. I think everyone in attendance, including me, would not be able to get ENOUGH of their messages. Well done, Rocco and Jennifer. I applaud you!

Lesson learned - You can choose your friends, but you cannot choose your family. That is God's decision. Trust Him. When God's purpose brings His children together, something amazing happens. They begin to discover how much love the human heart can hold. They begin to learn how far they can go spiritually, emotionally, and intellectually when the mode of travel is love.

# Chapter Fifteen

## MAKING IT WORK AND MAKING IT COUNT
### The Family Unit

---

*I do not want to get to the end of my life and
find that I have just lived the length of it. I
want to have lived the width of it as well.*

---

**DIANE ACKERMAN**

If you look up the word family in the dictionary, you will find several definitions. If you asked me for my definition of family, I would start by reiterating words I hear Rocco and Jennifer say every single day. "Call me if you need me," and "I love you." Rocco is always ready to lend a hand. Jennifer wants her final thought after goodbye to come from the heart. Work and love. You need them both to be a family. Love is not enough.

When one person in the family has autism, every person in the family has autism. We have two people in our family with autism. The impact intensifies. So how can we build some immunity against the toxicity of resentment? Reciprocity of unconditional love within a family is part of our DNA – we do not need to work at it – but mutual trust and respect are earned. Relationships take time and constant nurturing to become and remain fulfilling. Biology is simply the first date, the introduction. All too often, we take each other for granted. We are all guilty of this, and I am no saint.

Every human being has strengths and challenges. Yes, Domenico's and Roberto's autism is pervasive and all-consuming, but it cannot come first all of the time. Raising a family like ours takes staying power; it takes guts. We have found and continue to find ways to make accommodations in order to maintain an equilibrium that addresses the needs of every family member. Love is a good start. Love needs to be genuine and in constant supply. But day in and day out, it comes down to hard work.

We have tried. Gian and I have tried to make life as normal as possible for the six of us. We have hosted parties (Easter, Thanksgiving, Christmas). We have had barbecues with extended family and friends, just because. We have celebrated the children's birthdays (parties with their friends and parties with our family). All six of us have attended family get-togethers. All six of us have vacationed in Florida year after year for a ten-day stay. Gian and I have vacationed without the children several times (my parents moved in for the week). We have attempted going to mass on a regular basis as each of the children prepared for the sacraments of First Holy Communion and Confirmation. We have organized a Saturday craft night for quality family time. It would start with a game of bingo that engaged Domenico. He liked to spin the large, clear plastic ball that contained the small, numbered balls and match them to the template. We would then do a group activity such as painting. Maintaining Roberto's attention was challenging. We have enrolled all four children in swimming lessons (a life skill). Rocco wanted to learn how to play the guitar and Jennifer wanted to learn how to sing, so I drove them to the music academy. We created space in our house for the children. We had a room built adjacent to the kitchen for Domenico and Roberto. There, each has a comfortable armchair and they can watch a video on the television or listen to music on the CD player. We set up the basement with a television and sitting area for Rocco and Jennifer. When Jennifer was in secondary school, she moved into a larger, renovated bedroom in the basement. Rocco had already moved into his own bedroom in the basement a few years before. But as the years passed, life has unfolded in an atypical manner because of autism. We are not a normal family.

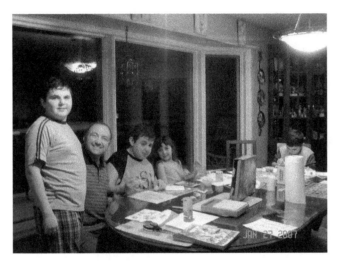

Craft night, January 27, 2007

I struggle at times with the realities of autism and the associated choices I have had to make. Would Rocco and Jennifer have explored other interests if I was in a position to involve them in activities like sports or the arts rather than having to stay home in order to maintain a predictable routine? If Gian did not have to shoulder the financial burden alone, could we have offered more opportunities for our children? I will, most certainly, carry this guilt for the rest of my life. The life lessons Rocco and Jennifer have gained from their brothers, however, have positively contributed to their development. I believe that with all my heart.

When Jennifer wrote, in a Mother's Day note, "You taught me that the best communication is when you do not use your words", I rejoiced! A standing ovation for Rocco who hugged me at day's end and said,

"Always remember that God is on your side." We remember one particularly challenging Thursday in May, as the bloodstained wall spoke to their brother's meltdown. Jennifer was crying, Domenico closed himself in the washroom, and Rocco stayed with Domenico while Roberto hit his head against the wall with all his might.

How do we, as a family, draw strength from the gifts of autism in the midst of its devastating reality? I will let you in on a little secret. There are four layers to our 'Happily Ever After' formula: clearly defining our roles, planning ahead, working together, and making sacrifices. The inevitable overlapping of these layers often results in roles playing out like sacrifices and planning ahead disguised as work.

*Roles.* Gian pounds the pavement outside of our house; I pound the pavement inside. Our roles are very traditional. This works for us. It may not work for you. Find out what works for you and commit to it.

I am home, full-time, with our four children. Gian leaves the house six days a week and puts in fourteen-hour days on the job. He is the sole breadwinner. Seems black and white, but it is not. While there needs to be autonomy within roles, these roles cannot flourish in isolation. What made the difference for us was a growing respect for and appreciation of the workload and stresses of the other. Having an understanding of what the other person's day entails requires ongoing and open communication. Simply asking how the other person's day was may not be enough. Get specific. Perhaps there can be a cross-over of responsibilities every now and then? Maybe, on a given day, you could help out. And maybe you could ask for help when you are feeling overwhelmed. There will be times in our lives when we provide for another's need, and other times when we are in need.

Gian's work commitments ease during the winter months. His hours are more nine-to-five. I remember the winter he taught Roberto to dress himself. I often do for Domenico and Roberto what they can do for themselves, sometimes because of time restraints, and sometimes because I cannot see them get it wrong. But Gian thinks more to their future independence (and has the strength to work for it). Gian would give Roberto an article of clothing and either verbally guide him or physically assist him in part. Roberto learned the skill of dressing that winter. When Gian's work hours expanded in the spring, I wanted to build on the advances they had made together. To this day, before Roberto starts dressing, I bring up a mental picture of me sitting on my hands so that I won't help him when he can do it for himself. But all too often, I dress him (please don't tell Gian).

Gian and I never wanted Rocco and Jennifer to provide the daily care for their brothers. We wanted them to enjoy as normal an upbringing as possible. They began with a few assigned household chores. As the years passed, Rocco and Jennifer have assumed greater responsibilities, but again, they were not responsible for their brothers. Every time I hear Rocco say, "It's the least I can do," after I ask him for a helping hand, I become almost giddy. He knows that Gian and I have assumed the daily care for Domenico and Roberto so that he is free to just be himself. And he appreciates it.

But what happens when Gian and I die, a hundred years from today? Rocco and Jennifer do not automatically become Domenico's and Roberto's legal guardians by virtue of lineage. It is a conversation we will need to have. I'm not ready to talk about it at this time. But perhaps the subject matter has already come up, without us saying a single word. On September 4, 2016, I was involved in a vehicular accident. An inattentive driver ran a red light, leaving me seconds away from a swift and painful death. Following the accident, Jennifer told me that she had considered the worst case scenario. If I had died or was incapacitated, she had a plan. She was prepared to lose a year of school to take care of her brothers. That's love at work.

Gian and I have talked about the day we are no longer here. It is our final hope to secure Domenico's and Roberto's future, long before we die. While we are still here, they will move into a group home. We will remain an integral part of their lives while giving them space to forge new and meaningful relationships. I will prepare visual schedules, social stories, and meatballs on demand (we love our meatballs). Gian and I will gradually come to know that they are in loving hands (we will feel it). If possible, we would like for Domenico and Roberto to live together. Funding for their needs will be approved and financially they will be self-sustaining. This is our sincere prayer. But should we be called to eternal life with unfinished business regarding Domenico and Roberto, Rocco and Jennifer will make it their business to honour our final wishes. They will step up to the plate and see our plan through to fruition. We know that.

As a unified team, Gian and I try to set a standard of excellence to inspire our children. We put forth our personal best for our children to emulate. If we afford them understanding, unconditional love, and support, perhaps they will too. If we lead by example, hopefully our children will follow.

*Planning ahead.* Autism does not do spontaneity. Autism does not do last minute changes. Autism plans ahead. We plan ahead. Planning is so vital to Domenico's and Roberto's well-being, that for their sake (if I could) I'd orchestrate my own death.

Our annual trip to Florida requires a lot of planning. We all look forward to it. We all work for it. The family condominium is our one hope for a successful vacation. A resort introduces too many changes. The cost of six flights to the Sunshine State exceeds our budget. We choose to drive. We choose to make the drive in twenty-four hours or less. After all, Domenico and Roberto would find no sleep at a hotel for an overnight stopover. We stop only to fuel up and to answer nature's call. We always leave on a Saturday morning at 8:30 a.m. Traffic is light, and the only delay is at the border. By 10:00 p.m., we are all wanting for some comfort food. We stop at a fueling station that is adjacent to a fast food restaurant. Not the healthiest choice, but warm French fries really hit the spot. We arrive in Florida the next day, close to the time we left, at around 8:30 a.m. Everybody feels spent, achy, and claustrophobic. But we arrive safely.

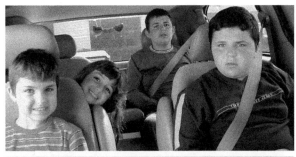

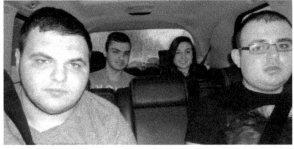

Driving to Florida over the years (2006 top and 2013 bottom)

Now we can start a no-agenda ten-day vacation, right? Not so fast. First we need to set up Domenico's and Roberto's visual schedules. That is my job. Someone needs to unload the car, and so Gian handles that. Rocco and Jennifer walk across the street and pick up some groceries to get us through the day. Domenico and Roberto take it all in and keep it all together. No one has a meltdown; no one is upset. They feel safe.

Morning walks, afternoon swims, the holiday itinerary is simple - just chill and let the good times roll. Autism speaks to its complexity and says, "Nice try." One year, we went parasailing. Domenico had his first seizure four hours later. Another year, Gian purchased a waterproof mP3 player for Roberto. Because he would tread water the entire time he was in the swimming pool, Gian wanted him to listen to some music. One day, Roberto pulled the wires off the headphones and broke the mP3 player. Three weeks later, we discovered that one earbud had remained in his ear. If not for the discharge coming from his ear, the bud may have stayed in longer. His doctor could not even see it when I brought him in for a check.

Autism does not take a vacation. The drive is hard. The days are structured. The routine is set in stone. It is not the dream vacation. Instead, it is precious family time that we crave, that we earn. That is what keeps us going back, year after year: our time together. I remember one drive home from Florida, more than a decade ago. Whatever virus joined us for the drive came out from both ends, with vomitus and diarrhea in heaps, times four children. I would barely finish with the clean-up of one spew only to start on the next. Squished between the rear seats of our minivan, nose deep in a gastrointestinal haze, I thought I was next. Gian offered to pull over so I could get some fresh air. I assured him that I was okay and to keep going. It was only another eighteen hours.

Our time in Florida is like hitting the 'refresh' button on life. As a family, we do things there that we rarely do at home. We enjoy simple stuff like playing cards or cooking meals together. Although it presents many changes for Domenico and Roberto, there is enough familiarity to comfort them. Domenico doesn't sleep the night before we leave for Florida as he is too excited. Roberto maintains a more cautious demeanour and at times is a hard read. I cannot conclude with complete certainty if he is happy by simply looking at his facial expressions. I need to assess his behaviour and ability to move from transition to transition (such as from the breakfast table to the washroom to the car the morning we leave). If he can do this with minimal stops to adjust something in this path like a chair for example, and is not vocalizing, I know he is in a calm and alert state. When both Domenico and Roberto smile, the universal language, I know they are in a good place.

We plan for our vacations. We accept our respective roles. We make it work.

*Working together.* Sometimes this means we break down a task into smaller parts and assign jobs. Sometimes this means we accept the task in its entirety and see it through to completion. For the most part, we carry our own. We do not leave for another what we can do ourselves. This is a common courtesy that should be extended to every human being. When we are faced with a situation that requires 'all hands on deck', however, we do not ask questions. We just get busy.

Domenico and Roberto both have a seizure disorder that is managed well under medication. Picture this. It was a regular day. It was 3:30 in the afternoon on a weekday. Gian was at work. Domenico, Roberto, and Rocco were home with me. Jennifer, who had just started grade nine, had remained at school to make changes to her schedule. I had my car keys in hand and was ready to pick her up. Domenico and Roberto were coming along for the ride. Then I heard sounds from the adjacent room. They startled me. I heard noises resembling falling household items. Domenico was having a seizure. As I ran into the room, I saw that his body was convulsing. His legs were about to give way. I caught him before he fell to the ground. I called out to Rocco who came running upstairs. Rocco called 911. Roberto watched in confusion from his glider.

When EMS arrived, things moved very quickly. Domenico was to be transported to the emergency department of the closest hospital. Who would go with him? Jennifer needed to be picked up from school. Rocco and Jennifer could remain at home alone, but not Roberto. Roberto could not sit in an emergency department for hours on end. Gian was an hour's drive away. Support from family was an hour away. The paramedic sensed my mounting anxiety. He gently asked me to join him in the hallway. There, I could not see Domenico. I could not focus on his vulnerability, lying there, an intravenous line already started. This kind professional then asked if I would consider having Rocco accompany Domenico to the hospital. While Domenico was being transported to the emergency department with Rocco there to support him, I could, with Roberto, pick Jennifer up from school. Once back home, I could arrange for child care. I could finish preparing dinner for Jennifer, Roberto, and the caregiver. Jennifer could answer any questions the caregiver would have. I could then join Domenico and Rocco at the hospital. Gian could meet up with us later at the hospital.

When I arrived at the hospital two hours later, Domenico was resting comfortably. Rocco provided me with an account of what had transpired – bloodwork, urinalysis, and discussions with health care providers. He handed me Domenico's Ontario health card, afraid he would forget. And then he said, "I'm hungry." Rocco had missed dinner.

In this extreme example, we all did what was required for a successful outcome. Teamwork prevailed.

*Making sacrifices.* The dinner table. From generation to generation, the dinner table continues to be a gathering place. For us, the dinner table is our boardroom and our playground. The dinner table is where stories are shared, solutions are found, bonds are strengthened, and memories are made. This is where tempers flare and laughter is the main course. And for us, the dinner table is also a place where we make sacrifices.

We have already talked about the choices I have made. Those choices could be considered sacrifices. But I am not the only one. Everyone in my family has given up, deferred, compromised, and made sacrifices. Any relationship worth fighting for involves some degree of give and take. Prioritize. Be patient. Have empathy. Work hard. Okay, in theory, this all makes sense. In practice, this takes work and love.

Check this out. In June, 2015 both Roberto and Jennifer were graduating from secondary school. Roberto had successfully completed a seven-year Planning for Independence Certificate Program, and Jennifer had completed a four-year secondary school diploma program. Rocco was turning nineteen in July of the same year. In Ontario, the legal drinking age is nineteen (he was ecstatic; me, not so much). Roberto would turn twenty-one two weeks later. Plan A was to applaud all these milestones at home with extended family - cake, food, tributes, laughter. But Roberto had just transitioned to day programming. Everything was new for him, and he was overwhelmed. A noisy party, albeit celebratory, would crush him. Plan B proved to be even better, believe it or not. Instead of a party, we did something very ordinary. Something we rarely do. We went out for dinner, just the six of us. What made it extraordinary was the preparation involved in making it a success. Call the manager of the restaurant to request permission to take pictures - check. Visit the restaurant and decide which table would be best (table 55, corner table, window seat, nothing behind us, minimal stimulation, direct exit if necessary) - check. Reserve our table for 5:30 p.m. (restaurant not crowded) - check. Prepare the social story - check. Pre-select menu to minimize waiting - check (soup for me, this was all I could stomach). Bring extra anti-anxiety medication just in case - check. Bring iPod Shuffle to listen to music during idle times - check. Bring a change of clothes (to remain in the car for dignity) - check. Pray, I mean drop down to your knees and beg - check. Thank God all day, leading up to dinnertime, for the opportunity to learn how to make it happen - check, check, and check. Prayer and preparation made it possible. No meltdown, no confusion, no surprises. The manager even gave us a gift card to be used towards the cost of dinner. He was moved by my explanation of the social story, how it helps Domenico and Roberto, how hard life is for them. He was surprised that I would go to such lengths for a simple dinner. His reaction surprised me. Preparing a social story to help Domenico and Roberto cope with change was not an option for me. It was Mirian's law.

It was more than a dinner for me. The actual meal was the last thing on my mind. This was an opportunity to find unparalleled joy in the most humble of places. The dinner was a chance to show God that I can be filled with His Holy Spirit during times of fear and struggle. Time and time again, I find beauty and strength in the grip of autism. My happiness was and continues to be my gift to God. It was not a five-star restaurant and I spent little time selecting my outfit. But I wore my Sunday best because with my husband and four children, it was a five-star milestone moment. The best accessory I wore that evening was the cross around my neck.

The greatest sacrifice every member of my family continues to make is adopting Plan B. Dinner at 5:00 p.m., snack at 8:00 p.m., bed at 9:00 p.m. No going out as a family on a Sunday evening, the day before a new week. No last minute decisions to do anything like a dinner out or a movie. No lazy, stay-in-your-pajamas-until-noon kind of weekend. Quiet voices before morning departure, quiet voices after 9:00 p.m. Quiet voices at the dinner table. Sometimes, you must curb your enthusiasm all day long. No drop in visits from family or friends. No telephone calls in the evening. As a family, we have built our lives within the framework of autism. We exercise self-restraint to the hilt. We fulfill our roles, we carry out our plans, we work hard, and we love hard. End of story.

My husband and I each carry a heavy load, and we have little time to compare notes. Our days are long and apart. Although we labour through our day independent of the other, we are driven by the same energy: the betterment of our children. We are on the same page. This form of interdependence is fundamental for longevity and fulfilment within our relationship.

We had dreams like everyone else. We had ambitions and hopes and an image of the family we were going to build together. Our children would reach milestones, pursue their interests, and make a life for themselves. We live a very different reality from those past dreams, and yet we still dream. We still hope and pray and work to be our best selves and to live our best lives despite the daily hardships and heartaches. Individually and as a team, we have triumphed because we believe in ourselves, in each other, and in God.

As often as possible, reflect on the reasons you decided to share a life with your chosen partner. Remind each other of what you wanted from life. If your dreams have been derailed, get back on track. If your expectations have been lowered, re-evaluate and raise them up again. If something is broken, fix it rather than throw it away. Sometimes, it is as simple as that, but at a minimum, it is the first forward step in actualizing the life you always wanted.

Sometimes you need more from life. Go get it. I love being Gian's wife. I love being a mother to my children. But these roles do not define me, nor are they enough for me. I want more out of life. My mouth is the biggest part of my anatomy, my ego is very small, but, all modesty aside, I have something to offer. So do you. You have a contribution to make.

Whatever may be going on at a given time in the lives of you and yours, try to be patient with each other. Focus on doing what is right, not wanting to be right. Help your significant other understand his or her own thoughts. Communication is more than just using your words. Effective dialogue involves choosing the right words and the right time to share them. The practice of understanding what is being said without making assumptions should be exercised as often as possible. Really listen. Ask questions for clarification. Receptive language is what we understand. Expressive language is what we say. I try to say what I mean and mean what I say. I try to walk the talk.

If every member of my family remains committed to the well-being of each other, we will all find our way in life. We will all reach our potential. When we labour with all our hearts for a common purpose, we define the family unit. Because that is what families do: they help each other, no matter what. And it works!

Lesson learned - Love is not enough; it all comes down to hard work. Sometimes the hardest part is deciding whether you love enough and want it bad enough to work for it, against all odds.

# Chapter Sixteen

## IN SICKNESS AND IN HEALTH

*Start calling yourself healed, happy, whole, blessed,
and prosperous. Stop talking to God about how
big your mountains are, and start talking to
your mountains about how big your God is!*

**JOEL OSTEEN**

Autism gave me the artillery to fight an enemy that had lain dormant in my psyche since January 3, 1986: my first date with Gian. That enemy was fear. Gian was born with an inherited disorder called Alport Syndrome. His mother also had the disease. It is progressive and leads to kidney failure in some. Renal transplantation is recommended for people facing end-stage kidney failure.

August 20, 1980 marks the day Gian received the gift of life, a second chance. It was a Wednesday, my favourite day of the week. His kidneys were partially working but failing rapidly when dialysis was recommended in May of that year. Dialysis would make him feel better. After four rounds of dialysis he described his quality of life as teetering just above the flat line, in other words, near death. Gian was admitted to the hospital one life-changing weekend for a Cystoscopy on Saturday, August 16. A Cystoscopy is a procedure used to examine the lining of the bladder and the urethra, the tube that carries urine out of the body. It was the evening of Sunday, August 17 when a doctor and a nurse entered his hospital room with good news. They asked Gian to guess. With the Cystoscopy complete, Gian thought he was going home. "Even better than that," said the doctor. "We have a kidney for you." A teenage boy from a vehicular accident had succumbed to his injuries. Gian's sixteen-year-old conscience begged the question: "How did my name sky-rocket to the top of the waiting list?" His doctor explained that because he was currently in the hospital, the same age as the deceased, relatively healthy (still passing urine), and the same blood type, he was the perfect match. Gian was the ideal candidate to receive this donor kidney. Following kidney transplantation surgery, Gian spent the next two months in the hospital.

Three decades later, Gian remembers his hospital stay with gratitude. My favourite story from his recovery is of a conversation between him and a nurse. One day, she walked into his hospital room and asked him why he was always smiling. Gian explained that he felt lucky to have received a kidney transplant. The nurse was bewildered. She could not understand his answer. She had expected him to be angry about why he had kidney disease in the first place.

Early into our relationship, I asked Gian how long his kidney would last. He said as long as he does. That was the first and last time we ever spoke about his health issues, at least out loud. Though never spoken about in any specific terms, we are both very cognizant that he is at risk. Every morning, Gian takes immunosuppressant medication. This is to ensure his immune system does not reject his transplanted kidney, a foreign organ. Compromising the body's natural defences in this way predisposes Gian to diseases such as cancer - the enemy. His mother, who had a kidney transplant one year prior to his, lost her battle with cancer on May 15, 1991. Developing life-threatening illnesses is a very real possibility for transplant recipients with weakened immune systems. Gian's mom would have celebrated her fiftieth birthday that June.

Gian developed basal cell carcinoma, a type of skin cancer, in 2007. Removal of these recurrent waxy bumps involved cauterization or freezing. These procedures were performed annually in the hospital's dermatology department. But they kept coming back, in different locations, all over his body. In 2013, Gian was diagnosed with squamous cell carcinoma, another form of skin cancer. Removal required day surgery. Also in 2013, Gian developed mouth sores and inflammation of his gums. We initially thought it was gingivitis that would flare up and subside in relation to the foods he ate and the beverages he drank, but in 2014, a biopsy confirmed pre-cancer cells in the lining of his mouth. In 2015 Gian had two surgeries, seven months apart, to remove the "bad cells". I was trying to prepare myself psychologically for what I feared was the inevitable. At age fifty, Gian was to follow in his mother's footsteps. I was convinced that this was the beginning of the end. At this point, autism became a friend and a teacher.

Just like autism, I am faced with another reality that I cannot change. Without the immune system to fight it, Gian could develop cancer or other devastating diseases. The pre-cancer cells in his mouth were very small. But my fear, that those cells would change, metastasize, and ultimately take his life, was very big. After crying an ocean of tears, I challenged myself not to let fear get the better of me. I took myself on. I wanted to prove to myself that autism had given me the skills to live through adversity. I wanted to believe that the pain of autism would bring about something good, as long as I did not quit. From the iron fist teachings of autism, I drew instruction on how to survive: Picture your life beautiful, Prepare to succeed, Take control of what you can, and Listen for the word of God in the silence of non-verbal autism.

*Picture your life beautiful.* My thoughts were heavy and dark. Gian's health was in question and I was panic-stricken. Autism had taught me to think in pictures. I wanted to surround myself with positive images. I made a collage with pictures of Gian, me, and our children. I posted this collage on the backsplash of my kitchen, the room where I spend most of my day. Every time I would look at our smiling faces, I would be reminded of the moment and the energy each picture communicated. Pictures are non-transient (Chapter 8). Unlike words, they will not go away. They will remain fixed, like the deep roots of a sheltering tree, to help me stand up to the threat of cancer. Using Boardmaker, I printed out copies of Psalm 23, the Lord is my Shepherd; and the Prayer of St. Francis of Assisi, Lord Make Me an Instrument of Thy Peace - my two favourite scripture writings. I superimposed these passages on separate images of a staircase leading up to a bright light. I committed them to memory and would recite them, like a mantra, during intervals of weakness and resolve. The vitality behind the words virtually became human, like a warm embrace. I also dug up some post-it note messages that I had saved. "Mentally strongest person I know" was a 2012 birthday tribute from Rocco. Jennifer wanted me to know that I was not alone when she wrote, "I prayed for you tonight." For their sake, I could not crawl under a rock and hide. I had to be present, mind, body and spirit. I typed out some words of wisdom and taped them close to the collage, post-it notes, and other pictures. Okay, since you asked, here are some of them:

> *Outside of the will of God, there is nothing I want.*
> *And within the will of God, there is nothing I fear.*

— A.W. TOZER

> *Life is a beautiful struggle.*

— UNKNOWN

> *Together, we can do anything.*
>
> — UNKNOWN

> *Family is everything.*
>
> — ROCCO

> *You are my home.*
>
> — JENNIFER

I read these messages over and over and over again, and I felt happy. I created for myself a visual oasis to wash away the depravity of fear and to hydrate my spirit. Similar to the affirmation page at the end of every social story, I was telling myself through pictures and words that *everything was going to be okay.*

*Prepare to Succeed.* Autism insists I always have a Plan B should Plan A fail. Do your homework, be prepared, always be one step ahead, pray, repeat, every single day when living with autism. That's my rule. But I did not want to prepare myself for the possibility that Gian would lose a battle with cancer similar to that of his courageous mother. Sinking into a deep-seated sadness faster than quick sand was not an option, but I wanted to. If their father became gravely ill, or for that matter if I fell ill, Domenico and Roberto would still have autism. The engine had to keep running. Life could not stop. I had to take my thoughts where I did not want them to go so that I could make peace with them. I had to get comfortable with what made me very uncomfortable: life without Gian. In order to understand myself and how I would achieve this mindset, I had to understand my thoughts. Self-awareness continues to be a prerequisite to living well with autism. I started a journal. Writing my fears down on paper somehow drained them of their power. The words, once bold and brazen, faded behind the lines on the pages like enemy forces surrendering. I made one entry in my journal on July 25, 2015: *I am afraid I am going to lose the love of my life.* I also started to write Gian's obituary. I had to. I had to be prepared to honour him. If the unspeakable happened, I would be too broken to find the words. I did it in such a way that kept him very much alive and well for decades to come. I left blanks. *To some of you, Gian was your employer; to others, he was your colleague, cousin, friend, son, son-in-law, brother, brother-in-law, uncle, to _____ he was your godfather, to ____ he was your father, and to one, he was the world, my world.* I wrote nothing further and have not expanded on this initial draft. I never went back to look at the words and the sentences. I just know where to find them, should I need to. Leaving space in the front of my journal for future entries, I then flipped to the back and started jotting down ideas for this book as they came to mind, as I lived them. I would be on a walk with Domenico and Roberto when my thoughts would beam me up to a higher consciousness. While exercising, I may have been stretching my muscles, but I was scarcely aware of my movements as I punched out a new reasoning. Writing this book, quite simply, has saved my life. This book you hold in your hands has helped me shift my obsession with death and disease, disability and despair, to God and love, purpose and personal growth.

*Take control of what you can.* I was terrified. Every day, my head would throb, my lungs would run laps, my chest would hurt, my belly would be in my throat, and my body would shake. I was consumed. The fear of the unknown, Gian's health, was swallowing me up whole. I had to do something. I set a goal to exercise a minimum of four times a week. I was pumped. I exercised five out of seven days the first week. Please do not be impressed. Some weeks, I scored a failing grade of two out of seven. I tried to forgive myself when the reason for not exercising was genuine, not an excuse. I went to visit our pastor after Gian's first surgery. I had met our pastor through Jennifer's involvement in the

youth programs offered at our parish. His smile is big and his love
for God is bigger. I knew I could talk to him. I told Father that I was
frightened, but not as much as I should be. That scared me. He told
me that I was already living the beatitudes of Jesus: "Blessed are the
poor in spirit, for theirs is the kingdom of heaven. Blessed are those
who mourn, for they shall be comforted. Blessed are the meek, for they
shall inherit the earth. And so on." A great sense of peace came over
me as I listened to Father's words. The fear, however, would return
in waves as the weeks of waiting for the second surgery turned into
months. I called a distress line on nine separate occasions. The first
thing I said was that I was not in crisis; I was not suicidal. The voice at
the other end of the telephone said, "That's good." These words were
oddly comforting to me. I explained that I just needed an objective
ear to hear me cry. The benefits of this intervention sustained me for
only a short while. I could not afford to see a counsellor at $160.00
per hour, but I needed someone to talk to on a more regular basis.
I found a centre for families that offered a sliding scale (adjusted to
one's financial resources), but there was a waiting list. I could wait.
Once there, my counsellor helped me understand that Gian's prognosis was good and to focus on his good health. I followed her advice.
She also recommended meditation. But even a brief three-minute
internet-guided session is hard to squeeze into my busy brain. I need
to schedule time for meditation and commit to it. Though I am sure it
will help, I am failing miserably.

The best thing I initiated to take control of my life was to highlight all
the positives. This was a mental exercise that, like any other training,
gets easier the more you do it and it actually became a good addic-
tion for me. I would think and think and think. This is what I came
up with: How lucky I am to have someone who makes the thought
of life without him unbearable. Read it over again; my mantra is a
little confusing. What good fortune to have found such a partner that
life without him is unspeakable. Gian and I do not have possessions
that would suggest success, but we have each other, and that is the

ultimate life acquisition. We are providing for our children and building a future. Because of autism, we cannot engage in adventures like a real vacation or other recreational activities as a family. Some days, we cannot even carry on a conversation in our own home, but we are happy and hopeful and working together. I have also made a point of telling my husband several times a day that I love him! Text messages, post-it notes, and telephone calls make it feel like the first date again.

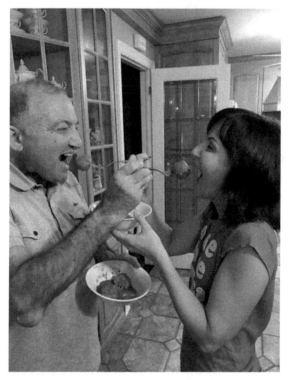

Twenty-eight years later and it still feels like the first date

*Listen for the word of God in the silence of non-verbal autism.* God wants us to come to Him with our troubles. He wants us to lean on His word when we are wandering or wanting. I listen for God's message and look for God's presence everywhere I go. Every time I pull into a crowded parking lot and find the best space vacant, I thank God.

When I turn the radio on and hear a song from the past playing, I thank God. That song takes me back to a happy time. Searching the internet for inspirational messages, I thanked God when I came across this one: "Someone asked God, 'If everything is already written in destiny, then why should we wish for something?' God smiled and said, 'Maybe in few places I have written, as you wish.'" When I am shopping and a pair of shoes magically flies off the shelf and lands on my feet, I take it as a sign from God that I should buy them. In the big things and the little things, God is there.

God comes to me through others. I just know it. I feel it. God knew my fears about Gian and understood my thoughts. One Monday morning, I was at the grocery store. Like every other day, I was deciding what to cook for dinner. Beside me, an elderly gentleman was doing the same thing. We were both looking for the best cut of meat. I noticed a small basket at his feet with a few food items in it. He seemed confused. I initiated some cordial conversation and was overcome by what he said. He told me that his wife of fifty-three years had just passed away. She had done all the cooking. He did not know how to cook. I assured him that cooking is easy. Start simple, was my advice. I helped him with his selection. He put the meat in his basket, thanked me, and left. It was the first and last time I ever saw him, but I think of him often and pray for him. I offer prayers for healing, prayers for peace. That was God in the grocery store, I am certain. God was telling me that life is hard, but to not be afraid. He will protect and provide. He will comfort and guide us through the darkness, into His light.

God also has a sense of humour. Bet you would have never thought so. Again, while waiting for Gian's second surgery, my worries would swell and deflate like the bellows of an overworked instrument. In the evenings Gian and I often fall asleep on the couch, wake up at around two in the morning, and then find our way to bed. One night I could not fall back to sleep. Although Gian crashed the minute his head hit the pillow, my thoughts kept me up. I started crying. Okay, I started sobbing. Okay, I started blubbering like a baby. I prayed Psalm 23 as I watched Gian sleep. Then he started to snore and I started to laugh. I laughed until it hurt, with tears in my eyes. I looked up and said, *thank you, God; I know that was you.*

We later learned those "bad cells" were squamous cell carcinoma, his second bout. Gian underwent a third surgery on March 21, 2016 to remove the cancer. It was life-changing (long story, happy ending, next book). The silent world of autism has amplified God's message and His voice and I am clinging to every word.

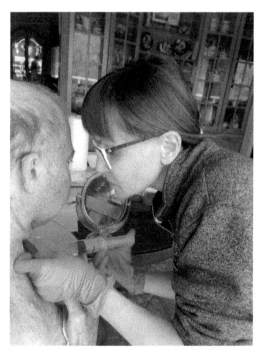

I always wanted to be a nurse. Irrigation to treat
infection following March 21, 2016 surgery

I married a man with kidney disease. What did I expect? Did I expect to go through life without seeing the inside of a hospital room? If I had answered "yes", I would be deeply ashamed of myself. It would be selfish of me to want a euphoric existence while the rest of humanity endures its rations of misfortune. No, I did not expect life with Gian to read like the pages in a romance novel. But I also did not expect to grow strong in the broken places because of our love. I did not expect to fall in love with the same man over and over again in a twenty-eight-year love affair (and counting). I did not expect our love to survive two diagnoses of autism for over two decades (and counting). Love has been a faithful and discerning force, a friend, and a teacher. Love is stronger than fear.

Lesson learned - Lean on God, the Father of love, in good times and in bad, in sickness and in health. Let your reliance on God be greater than that of any human, including you. His love is complete. All you need is His love.

# Chapter Seventeen

## A FATHER'S LOVE

*My father gave me the greatest gift anyone
could give another person: He believed in me.*

**JIM VALVANO**

My husband once said, "They will go wherever we take them." He was referring to Domenico and Roberto. He was speaking of their dependency and vulnerability. And it scared me, but he was right.

Okay, enough of me and my big mouth. I do not know about you, but I am a little tired of hearing my own voice. Would you consider spending some quality time with my husband Gian?

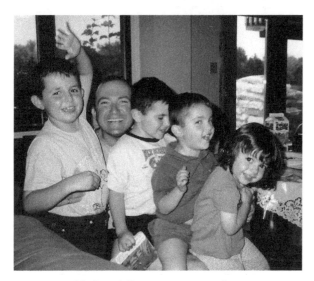

All aboard, Row, row, row your boat

Behind a quiet confidence lies a man of massive character. A learned man, highly regarded, this professional engineer's crowning accomplishment is his vision. Renal transplant recipient of thirty-seven years strong and an eight-time participant in the Enbridge Ride to Conquer Cancer, Gian has $208,000 to his fundraising name.

Gian approaches life with the mindset of a scientist. He applies the principles of mechanics, design, and chemistry to help organize his world. Gian knows his way around the Periodic Table of Elements, but when it comes to love, he's all heart: he is the noble element.

Welcome to the core of a father's love.

*What did you imagine fatherhood would look like?*

> I thought fatherhood would include an abundance of time with my children. I envisioned my kids following me around and participating in whatever task I was engaged in. That is what I hoped for. That is what I had with my dad, and I wanted to

experience the same with my children. The responsibilities of fatherhood, however, compounded by the additional weight of autism, are what follow me around. My idea of being a parent has changed from my initial belief. I have come to understand that primarily, fatherhood is my God-given task to protect and provide, and to model and mold a strong moral character in my children. I need to help them develop skills for life. And that is the reality. That is the truth. All four of my children are in this world in part because of me. I am committed to ensuring they find their way in the world. And I will not rest until that happens.

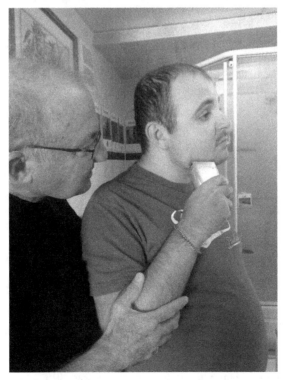

Gian teaching Domenico how to shave

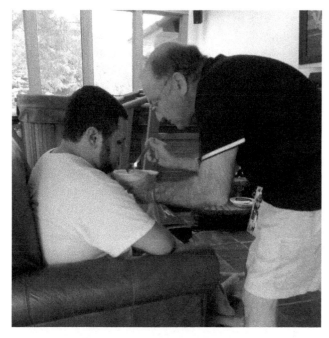

Gian sharing his lunch with Roberto

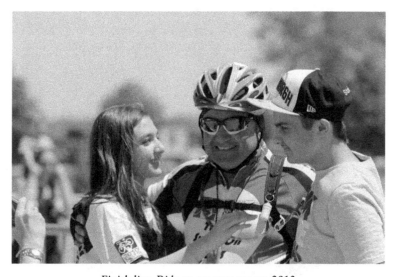

Finish line, Ride to conquer cancer, 2013

*How has autism impacted your life's goals and aspirations?*

I wanted a partner in life with whom I could raise a family to call my own. I wanted to start new traditions while observing those from years past. I wanted my children to grow with the times while bringing back the days when a handshake was enough. I wanted to provide for them financially, emotionally, and spiritually in a way that allowed enough space for their development. I wanted so much. Over the years, however, I discovered that what I really want from life is quite basic and quite absolute. I just want my children to be happy and to be able to share in that happiness! My sons' autism has shaped my life's goals and aspirations into more valuable ones. I learned that every stage in life can elicit real joy, even when hardships are constant.

Accepting that my sons will <u>never</u> have a normal life has allowed me to focus on what brings <u>them</u> happiness and hence steer their lives in that direction. Because of them, I have been able to truly appreciate the differences in others and 'see' how everyone contributes to this world in their own way. Because of them, I work harder to be kind, to be a friend, to empathize, and to give more. My goals and aspirations are aligned with those of my sons: to do the best I can and to be the best person I can be despite the circumstances that surround me.

*If you could snap your fingers and make their autism go away, would you?*

For my sons' sake, I wish I could snap my fingers and make their autism go away. I fear for their future when the day comes that I can no longer care for them. Like any parent, I worry that my children will suffer in my absence. For my sake, however, I do not want for the abolishment of autism. Domenico's and Roberto's strengths and challenges have enriched my life. They have helped me become more aware of the needs of others (whatever those needs may be) and more tolerant of those needs whether I can understand them or not. Domenico's and Roberto's autism has allowed me to witness compassion and acceptance in our society in ways that I otherwise may not have seen.

*When you think of your future, what does it look like?*

I see my future being similar to that of many parents. The dependence of my younger children on me will diminish as they learn to care for themselves. Domenico's and Roberto's independence will take more time. Retirement will need to be deferred. Residential placement for Domenico and Roberto will need to be considered. I will have to continue to take a leadership role in fostering their growth as valued members of society through awareness, integration, and active participation with others. I will never stop being their dad.

*What advice would you give to parents just receiving a diagnosis of autism?*

My advice to any parent receiving a diagnosis of autism for his or her child is to be prepared to give and <u>show</u> as much love as possible to your child. Integration in society has and continues to be the most positive avenue in their lives. Achieving true integration, however, takes tremendous and ongoing effort through a leadership role from preschool to adult programming to residential placement.

Perseverance is key as you will encounter many setbacks which can be discouraging. Your positive energy is critical in motivating others to work as hard as you do towards the success of your child. Believe in your child's ability as you would any other child. Celebrate his or her achievements, however small, in a big way. Let him or her know how awesome you think he or she is, every single day. The rewards are immeasurable. A smile from my children is all it takes to elevate my spirit to tremendous heights. A hug from my children can melt away the sorrows of any day. I can sit in the complete silence of non-verbal autism with my children and feel that I just had the best conversation of my lifetime. And when I hold their hands, I know I have the whole world in my hands.

*How brilliant is your wife? Rhetorical question, Gian; no need to elaborate. That would take all day.*

Gian and I were not ready to be parents. Financially, we were not on solid ground. Professionally, we were just starting. Emotionally, we were immature. In terms of life experience, we had little to prepare us for autism. But we had each other. And we knew what we wanted. We wanted a family. We cannot define parenthood in words. We can only live it. We live it as if each and every day is a privilege. Every day, I see that Gian is more than a father, he is a dad.

Lesson learned - Fatherhood is more about the child than it is about you. It is more than throwing the first ball. More than the hero's welcome every night to fill your void. More than having a miniature version of yourself to illuminate your life. It is about you lighting the path for your child to find his or her own way. It is about being there, all there, regardless of the overtime. It is about loving someone more than you love yourself. "It is about you, because if it is about you - Domenico, Roberto, Rocco, and Jennifer - then it is about me too."

# Chapter Eighteen

## THE GIFTS OF AUTISM

*Comfort and prosperity have never enriched the world as much as adversity has done. Out of pain and problems have come the sweetest songs, the most poignant poems, the most gripping stories. Out of suffering and tears have come the greatest spirits and the most blessed lives.*

**BILLY GRAHAM**

Where do I start? The gifts of autism are boundless. You cannot count them on your fingers. You cannot measure them on a scale. If you are shaking your head in disbelief, I don't blame you. What good could come from a lifelong disability that seems to only take, deplete, and extinguish? We already touched upon the gift of self-awareness in Chapter 12. Here are four more reasons to believe that from unrelenting pain comes unparalleled joy: The Gift of Ministry, The Gift of Humanity, The Gift of Peace, and The Gift of Hope.

*The Gift of Ministry:* We all have talents and skills to offer. We all have experiences and insights to share. In our daily labour, in the service we provide, in the circumstances we endure, we are all teachers and students alike. Many people involved in Domenico's and Roberto's lives over the years have ministered to me. Three members of the school team thought they were just doing their job. I know that they were doing God's work. Their counsel positively impacted how I live with autism to this day. They gave me words I will never forget.

This too shall pass: Domenico, in his elementary school years, used to wander from home. Whenever neighbours would burn waste in their backyards, Domenico's curiosity took him there. One time, he was returned to me by a neighbour like a piece of garbage that had spilled onto her lawn. She knew why he had trespassed, or so she said, and she knew what I was going through. I questioned her ability to understand what was involved in parenting a child with autism. But I did not even know. I just knew I had a problem to solve. I e-mailed a school board appointed autism specialist for advice. Suggestions included spray painting a line on the lawn as a "do not enter" visual reminder. I could take a picture of Domenico standing on our side of line, prepare a one-page visual, and reinforce the expectation before he went outside. At the end of this specialist's e-mail, he typed out four golden words, "This too shall pass." I took this assurance to heart. Living with autism will be mapped with challenges and setbacks. I have to remain calm in my heart. If I allow every negative experience to bury me, I will face a swift, inner death. Adopting an emotional shield against intolerance and misunderstanding was imperative for survival.

A wonderful conversation: There is a difference between communication and talking with words. I know that now. We speak volumes with what we do not say with our words. Non-verbal forms of communication such as gestures require our ability to understand their meaning. One day, a speech and language pathologist spent some time with Domenico in order to consult with the school team. She later told me that they had shared a wonderful conversation. She was referring to Domenico's communicative attempts - behaviour, vocalizations, facial expressions, body language, eye contact, and overall demeanour.

This was a pivotal shift in the way I interacted with Domenico and Roberto from that day forward. My sadness that they are non-verbal was replaced with an understanding that they still have a voice. I had to learn to read what they were saying with their eyes, with their actions, and with their behaviours, within the context of their day. I am constantly watching them to keep the conversation going. Before, I hadn't known they were so chatty. I had thought I was the only one in the family with a big mouth.

I keep him guessing: Helping a person with autism become more adaptable to the unknown requires foresight and support. One educator had a strategy to help her students learn that life will not always follow a predictable routine, and that's okay. Domenico, who develops rituals specific to people, could not figure her out. She kept changing her ways - the order in which the school day unfolded, the materials used, the tasks completed - she kept him guessing. He could not attach a behaviour to a time or activity. As a result, his obsessions remained relatively quiet. I learned that although people with autism need stability, they also need spontaneity. This educator's example gave me the courage to introduce change. I had to strike a balance.

If you evaluate your interactions on a daily basis, you too have helped others. You too have received guidance. Regardless of the resources we have, the office we hold, or the conditions we live under, we should all reach out and share our knowledge. You never know the life you will change.

*The Gift of Humanity:* We are all human. We all have strengths and challenges. Nobody can claim world domination over life in all its ambivalence. Nobody has all the answers. Life is frail and fragile, complex and forever changing. Within our relationships and daily interactions, there needs to be room for personal expression, human error, and genuine empathy. A person with autism brings other people together in a very cohesive and intimate manner. This is particularly true in school, work, day programs, and residential settings.

The strengths and vulnerabilities of all team members need ongoing validation and support. Everybody demonstrates behaviours that could be considered autistic and potentially problematic. I am very precise when it comes to time. I remember calling a doctor's office because I was late for my appointment. It was 10:03 in the morning. My appointment was scheduled for 10:00. The first thing I do in the morning is make the bed, even if Gian is still sleeping in it. All labels on cans and boxes need to be facing forward. Gian will forget to take his medication in the morning if his routine is altered. He needs all doors to be fully opened or completely closed. When we host dinner parties, Gian sketches out a seating plan as well as placement of dishes on the buffet table. He is a visual thinker. What's even more disturbing about this behaviour is that after years of marriage, I started doing the same thing. Jennifer needs her bedroom furniture to be perfectly aligned. Wall and floor tiles that do not follow a linear pattern make her uneasy. While driving, Rocco sets the volume to thirteen when listening to the radio and twenty when listening to his music. A setting to an uneven number, in this case, thirteen, will trouble Jennifer if she rides with him (actually this will drive her crazy). Even numbers always have a pair and just make sense to her. When watching a YouTube video, Rocco will pause on an even number. Rocco likes to see a manicured lawn. If he is unable to trim the perimeter of our property, his concentration will be compromised all day long. Like Domenico and Roberto, we do not want to engage in these obsessive tendencies or recurring thoughts. But sometimes, we simply cannot stop ourselves. We need our family and our friends to understand and love us despite our idiosyncrasies. What a beautiful world we would live in if we welcomed diversity. Our world would be massive and magnificent, fascinating and enlightening. Let's be real in our hearts, in our minds, in our intentions. Let's help each other live out our personal and collective aspirations. What better way to love God than to love one another for who we are.

*The Gift of Peace:* I do not simply parrot the sacred writings of scripture, I truly believe. God, He is the creator of all, provider of all. Peace is not the absence of fear. Peace is the presence of God. He is everywhere, in the full rainbow of our happiness and in the dark shadows of our insecurities. He shares in our joys and in our sorrows. One day, I said His name out loud. Domenico and Roberto had joined a group for a four-day, three-night cottage getaway as part of a summer camp program. Rocco and Jennifer both had part-time employment. They tried to coordinate their schedules to ensure one of them would be home with me for the three evenings that Domenico and Roberto were away. They did not want me to be alone for dinner. Touched by this gesture of love, I reassured Rocco and Jennifer that I am never alone. God is with me! First, last, and all the spaces in between, God is there.

I feel a great sense of serenity every time I place myself at the centre of adversity and emerge victorious. Avoidance and denial that a problem exists will not make it go away. Facing our difficulties and living through our challenges builds character and skills for life. Knowing that God is already on the other side of pain, waiting, arms extended like a pathway to healing, helps me find my way. For me, peace is only possible with God. It takes a conscious commitment to build trust in God, believing His intention is greater than our discomfort. Accepting everything He sends as an opportunity to grow closer to Him is a promise I have made to God. My faith is stronger than my fear.

*The Gift of Hope:* I was at both ends of hope, wanting to give and needing to receive. I thought hope was easy to find, easy to exchange, and easy to uphold. I was wrong.

When Domenico and Roberto were in secondary school, I was asked to talk to a new parent whose son was recently diagnosed with autism. I jumped at the chance to highlight Domenico's and Roberto's gains and how much I had learned. I offered to help create a visual schedule and other supports. I invited her to my home where I could show her all the materials I had made for Domenico and Roberto. I gave her my contact information and looked forward to meeting her. I wanted the gifts of autism that I had experienced to be projected onto her. I thought I was offering her hope and encouragement. I later learned that I had conveyed too much optimism, too much positivity. She needed to talk about the emotional turmoil and inevitable hardships of autism. She needed time to process the realities of the diagnosis before she could take on the added responsibilities. I can only hope that in time, her pain has lessened and her joy has doubled.

With Domenico's transition to plan for, I sought advice from one parent whose son already attended a day program. I wish I had never made that call. I wish I had never engaged in that conversation. This parent had little but misery to offer. In her opinion, there were few day programs in the area and the one her son attended was mediocre. Having now gone through the process twice, I would deliver a different message to parents. I would recommend they visit the day programs themselves to get a vibe of the place and the people. I would assure them that there are several programs available and many dedicated people who want to help. I would never foretell a descent into despair. How are we to navigate our way through life if we do not have hope?

Life is not complicated for me. It is always the right time to do the right thing for my family, for my community, for myself, and especially for God. Anyone can minister to the needs of others, including me, including you. We do not need to possess unlimited funds to contribute to a cause, unrestricted access to resources is not necessary to lend a hand, showcasing the hardware of a decorated athlete is not a prerequisite to becoming someone's hero, and a single word does not even have to be spoken for our messages to be heard. We just have to care. We just have to want to make a difference. I want to make a difference. No doubt you want to make a difference too!

The gifts of autism are in all of us to give and take. Find those jewels that shine through you and you alone. Look for that unique luster in your neighbours and let's build a better future. If we consolidate our skills, if we remain true to ourselves and one another, if we work tirelessly for peace, and if we elicit hope above all, together, we could change the world.

Lesson learned - Autism is the gift that keeps giving. The lessons and the positive changes that occur when living through hardship will bring us closer to God. Every challenge is like the rung of a ladder in the climb to a better life: a life with God. That is the greatest gift of all.

# Chapter Nineteen

## PIECES OF MY FAITH

*And she always had a way with her brokenness. She would take her pieces and make them beautiful.*

**R.M. DRAKE**

Autism and faith are good friends, soul sisters, best bros. Did you know that? It's true. Not everybody believes in God, and that's okay. I do. With all my heart, I believe.

What is faith to you? To me, faith is having an audience with God, and making communication with Him a daily priority. There is an inherent degree of doubt in one's faith. Within that uncertainty lie the teachings of God's word. From these instructions the opportunity arises to glorify God's name by living according to His charge. Faith requires patience and time for life to unfold according to God's plan. And to do so, emphatically!

Shortly after receiving Domenico's diagnosis, I had a conversation with a parent of a child with autism. She was a veteran. Her son at that time was Domenico's age today. Twenty years have passed and I still remember her words. For her, living with autism was like living with the death of the child she thought she had given birth to, and experiencing that loss over and over again. I still pray for her today for she is surely in a dark place.

For me, autism has been the birth of light and hope, courage and opportunity, love and faith, twenty-five years strong. Yes, autism shattered my heart into a million pieces. Life as I knew it changed in an instant, so I started to gather those pieces, to be whole again.

Autism is mysterious and confusing, innocent and interesting, unique and honest. The international symbol for autism is an interlocking, multi-coloured puzzle piece to highlight the complexity of the disorder. Advances in understanding this perplexing condition have been made, and yet there are missing pieces to the puzzle. Professionals who study autism and families who live autism have many unanswered questions.

Living with autism is like working on a puzzle for the rest of your life without knowing what the image is or if you will ever finish the puzzle. The pieces are all different sizes, shapes, and colours and you have to fit them together. As you find new pieces, you discover that those already placed in the puzzle have disappeared. Now imagine assigning a word to each puzzle piece: words like acceptance, understanding, compassion, and respect. Each word has a story and a face. Then there are other words that should never be spoken, or lived. They exist. Discrimination, ignorance, exclusion, and denial are real. After two decades of living with autism, I came to understand that I was actually putting together the pieces of my faith. I want to be an autism advocate and a defender of faith. They go hand in hand.

When Domenico and I received a diagnosis of autism, it was as if God was in the room with us. I imagined Him there. As the doctor's words hung in the silent space of dismay, I visualized God handing me a box. It was unwrapped and plain looking. Once home, I dropped to my knees, removed the lid, turned the box upside down, and emptied its contents all over the floor. God had given me a puzzle, with the instructions missing. Bits and pieces of life and faith, autism and altruism carpeted the room like a human tapestry.

Come, kneel down with me. Let's talk about all the pieces I have gathered over the past twenty years. Let's put them together and see what we discover. I always look for all four corners and pieces with flat sides whenever I start a puzzle.

Acceptance and denial are elements of life that propel us forward or hedge us in. *Acceptance* of people with autism makes up all four corners and pieces with flat sides to frame the puzzle. No mystery there. Acceptance allows those with disabilities to live *outside* of the margins. Acceptance supports an inclusive society.

Within the family unit, peer group, or social circle, at different times we may encounter the welcome mat or the closed door. The relationships and circumstances we find ourselves in can be a birthright, an earned privilege, a harsh reality, or an unfortunate series of events. To be accepted for who we are and grow outward is a basic human need and a gift. God created us in His perfect image, to exalt our unique yet collective abilities, to live in harmony, to work side by side, and to love one another.

Not all classrooms, community centres, day programs, health care settings, work places, and other organizations we encountered have opened their doors and their minds to autism. The school-to-home communication book's only entry one day was an instruction to cut Domenico's fingernails. The community swimming pool had no family change room. The laboratory made no accommodations for those who struggle to sit in one spot for any length of time in order to wait their turn. The theme park did not have backdoor access for those with disabilities. The movie theatre did not have sensory-friendly viewing times when the lights are dimmed and the volume is lowered. Day Programs A and B did not accept Domenico because they claimed it would be too much work to support him (Chapter 9).

Denial into Program A, however, remains the darkest piece of the autism puzzle to date, with a story that needs to be told. I will never forget that one Friday in the fall of 2012.

Program A is organized into three subsets: The Woodery Woodworking Shop, The Craft Studio, and the Day Program. People are offered work and recreational opportunities in accordance to their abilities and interests. One work experience caters to artisans while another attracts those who enjoy working with wood. The day program engages people in diverse activities. I could see Domenico actively participating in any of the three.

I arranged to visit Program A on the first Professional Activity Day (P.A. Day) of the school year on Friday, September 14, 2012. As you read on, please remember the day of the week, Friday. It is relevant. Students do not attend class on P.A. Days. On Domenico's final year of secondary school, I did not want him to miss any school days to visit prospective day programs. Missing school would be too disruptive to his routine. As it was also a P.A. Day for Roberto, the three of us were given a tour of the grounds and the buildings by the program coordinator.

We first visited the Woodery. The group, focused on the task at hand, grinded to a halt upon our arrival. All drills and machinery were silenced. Everyone in attendance, prompted by the leader and other support workers, gathered around us. Before entering the building, the program coordinator had assured me that, as a newcomer, I would not be able to identify participants from support workers. She took pride in the community feeling. She called the participants the "core people" of the program. I liked that.

Jim, the leader, initiated an interactive and informative discussion of what the Woodery was all about. His explanation lasted ten minutes. Domenico's curiosity had him wandering into his own discussion and adjacent rooms. This is what he always does. Every time we visit a new place or return to a familiar setting, Domenico first orients himself by going from room to room, opening drawers and closets. He touches nothing, just looks, so that he can be comfortable with his surroundings, and so that he understands. Instead of standing to listen as the leader spoke, Domenico walked around. He wanted to know what was on the other side of the door and around the corner. Roberto, who finds a comfort zone wherever he goes, stood frozen by my side and *heard* the leader talk. Someone who does not know Roberto would have assumed that he was listening and understanding and that Domenico was not listening, not understanding, and not cooperating.

We were then guided through The Craft Studio and Day Program. At the tour's completion, I thanked the program coordinator for her generosity of time. An immediate drop down menu in my brain's computer had Domenico trialling the Woodery shop while Roberto was in the Craft Studio. The program coordinator explained that someone would have to accompany both Domenico and Roberto on that day. I would be that person. When she further elaborated that a training period was required before a candidate could be considered for acceptance into the program, I decided to focus my attention on Domenico solely. I would find someone to support Roberto on that day while Domenico and I were at the Woodery. I was excited and committed to Domenico's success. He would excel at this job. Promising to accommodate their schedule, I asked the program coordinator if I could come two weeks before the trial day to take pictures. I would prepare a social story and visual scripting for the trial. She agreed that this plan could work.

When I returned home, I e-mailed her to confirm the date that Domenico and I could trial the Woodery. I had suggested the second P.A. Day of the year. This was her reply, and I quote: "Following the tour, Jim did express a concern that Domenico did not stay in one place or listen to what the job would be like for him. I know from Jim's perspective that he may be most concerned with safety and also if Domenico would be able to work in a somewhat independent manner throughout the work day." The infamous safety parameter nauseates me. I have heard this excuse a million times. Her words hit me like a discriminatory slap across the face. I still turn red, every time I think about it. The workshop's leader had appointed himself judge, jury, and executioner after a brief ten-minute introduction to Domenico.

A futile e-mail exchange with the program coordinator followed. I made it easy for her to be less than honest with me. I told her that the one and only day I could support Domenico for his first training session was Friday, November 16, 2012, the next P.A. Day. My transparency helped me see through her hypocrisy. She assured me that she would follow-up with Jim regarding a trial of the Woodery. On September 27, she sent me a hollow e-mail reassurance that, although inundated with other commitments, she had not forgotten about us. By this point, I had dismissed her. She was biding her time and her words. She had no intention of allowing Domenico to trial the Woodery.

Her final e-mail of October 19 was very fluffy and pretty. She even used the word love. Let me know if you find an ounce of integrity in her message: "I hope this finds you and your family well. I am writing to inform you that the Woodery is unable to offer Domenico a trial on a Friday on the basis that we fundamentally do not offer trials or tours on Fridays. (I take full responsibility for the fact that I should not have changed that when I offered your family a Friday tour!) People in our work programs work very hard all week to get to Fridays, which is a day of celebration and a break from the business and many requests from our community. I understand the fact that the P.A. Day would be the most suitable day for your son but I do need to consider the needs of the individuals in the Woodery as well. Please know that I have given this a great deal of consideration and I truly am interested in learning much more about Domenico as well as Roberto. I have some ideas and would love the chance to talk when you have the time." Blah, blah, blah, how offensive. She did not even give Domenico a chance to fail. What an insult to his potential. What a mockery of the program's mission statement. I did not reply. Instead, I printed her e-mail and laminated it. I taped it to my desk, so I could see it every day, and remember. One year later, I received an e-mail from the manager of another day program. He was responding to my request for a meeting. Domenico was to start at the day program the next month. I had some questions and an introductory package for him and the support workers. His e-mail message was one of encouragement, affirmation, and genuine interest. I printed this affirmation, laminated it, and taped it on top of the other e-mail. This way, I could focus on the positive. Partiality, unfairness, and exclusion are not pieces of the autism puzzle.

We share the same space on planet Earth, but we do not all morph into the same sphere. Accommodations need to be made. Evolution is infinite. What if, more than accepting our differences, we embraced them? What if we tried to understand them? Our world will be so big, our lives so beautiful, if we learn how others do the same thing we do, but in a different way. We will all be stronger.

Perhaps the day programs that built a wall of ignorance to keep Domenico out have since made a door to let others in. Today, Domenico's and Roberto's needs are triaged for blood work and other laboratory tests to minimize the wait and the anxiety. Many community centres that I now visit have family washrooms and change rooms. Some educators have asked for a copy of my school-to-home communication system. Domenico and Roberto have been invited to a few movie theatres that offer sensory-friendly viewing times. Progress has been made. Autism awareness delivers an unequivocal message that together, we can build a better world, one piece at a time.

We need to further our understanding that we all belong. Denial and intolerance of our differences are barriers that need to be torn down.

Educating others about autism is an awesome and ongoing responsibility. Everyone invested will thrive. Let's frame our world with hope and help, open minds and open hearts. Just think of the possibilities.

Okay, we have the outer edges of the puzzle: *acceptance* into societal groups, programs, and services. Let's now strengthen the foundation of the puzzle with *faith*. We cannot go it alone in life. We need God's wisdom to pick up where ours leaves off.

Acceptance in autism is not limited to creating an inclusive society by ensuring accessibility, funding, and equity. It extends beyond our noble intentions as a people, far and away from our collective abilities, to God's covenant and supreme capability. Acceptance takes *faith*.

Roberto has memorized the location of his seat in known settings but needs to be reminded to put his shirt on the right way. Domenico can use his tablet to advance from track to track on his playlist but cannot colour within the lines. Domenico's obsession with hangers may preoccupy him from morning to night at times and then fade as if it never existed. Roberto may be worried about a loose thread on a towel and consequently rip it to shreds, but the hole in his shirt will go unnoticed. Why? All the grey areas of autism and life have taught me to have *faith*, to lean heavily on the wisdom of The Shepherd rather than being fenced in by my own discerning. He is an awesome God. He has all the answers.

Had I known at the time of diagnosis what I know now, I would have given up on autism. Domenico is able to trace a dotted line to print his name. He can copy a prewritten message onto a greeting card. In grade one I initiated a routine of having Domenico print the date every morning. This would improve his fine motor skills and teach him about the days of the week, or so I thought. I tried everything I could think of to encourage legible penmanship. I introduced different writing instruments (pencil, pencil crayon, marker, scented marker, fine point pen, medium point pen). I changed the booklet for the daily entries (traditional notebook, artist sketch pad, daily planner). I thought if I changed the orientation of the page from portrait to landscape, it would make a difference. I asked Domenico to write over my entry of the date (solid lines, dotted lines, missing letters, and highlighted letters). But Domenico's printing of the date never advanced beyond that of a preschool child. On April 2, World Autism Awareness Day 2015, I decided that December 31 of the same year would mark the end of this exercise and the start of peace, nineteen years later. For almost two decades, God had carried this painful reality for me. As the day approached, my excitement grew. I was not giving up; I was letting go. I was free, liberated. I could now focus on reaching greater heights that would applaud Domenico's strengths.

*Faith* involves active participation in the process of acceptance. Faith takes patience and a desire to learn about God as we wait for His lessons to be revealed and realized. We cannot understand everything that happens to us, all at once. Our station in life, the people who come and go at different times, are the writings of a human history book, with God holding the pen. Some people He sends into our lives to teach us, others He sends for us to teach. God wants us to gravitate towards those who do not quite fit in, and help them find their place. More than simply accepting diversity, when we follow God's example, when we adopt a "why not in my backyard" mindset, we build *compassion*.

Let's now look for the inner pieces of the autism puzzle. Let's look for *compassion, understanding,* and *respect*.

*Compassion* is a concern for the sufferings of another and a longing to ease their pain. It is a crucial piece of the autism puzzle and should be a part of our daily interactions. There is an assumption that those who enter the health care profession are driven by a desire to help and heal. A sense of social responsibility cannot be learned in the formal sense. One's "bedside manner" comes from within.

One doctor was driven by greed, another by grace. Dr. Spineless had two faces: caring and competent on the outside, self-serving and shallow on the inside. Domenico and I were in his office for our annual check-up. I asked him for a renewal of our prescription. His evasiveness confused me, as he instructed me to call the prescription in to his office when I returned home. This made no sense to me. I was in his office. Why could he not simply have provided the prescription renewal right then and there? I could see the prescription pad on his desk. One week following the appointment, I received a letter in the mail from his office. An annual fee would cover the cost for services, including prescription renewals. We needed the prescription then. He needed the annual fee moving forward.

I would have paid Dr. Spineless had he given me the prescription during that appointment. I had observed that he often rushed us through like cattle with little time for our questions. His refusal to refill our prescription in his office was the final stab in the back. I never saw him again. There was no room in our lives for his ego.

I have known Dr. Selfless for a decade now. He always ends our telephone consultations with a sincere, "It is my pleasure." Living in another country for two months at a time, his compassion travels to every region of our hearts. He has written countless letters in support of inclusion, completed endless forms required for community supports, and provided sound medical advice during the most difficult of times. I never received an invoice for his great efforts. The impact he has had on our lives is immeasurable. In truth, the pleasure and the privilege have been all ours.

*Compassion* and *understanding* need to be ever present in all our relationships, especially within the family. In Chapter 15, we shared a conversation about what it takes to raise a family while living with autism. It's a lifelong climb. Sometimes it takes remembering, so you continue to learn; and sometimes it takes forgetting, so you never give up. Sounds confusing, I know. Autism is complicated.

People with autism need a predictable routine, yet within that sameness, they demonstrate different behaviours at different times. *Understanding* that some of their behaviours may never be reasoned or resolved requires *compassion* and *faith*.

I do not remember how old Roberto was when it happened. But at one point his obsessions would not let him sleep...not let him sleep... NO SLEEP. The story of the wake-up call dates back to elementary school. The glass fragments, the broken picture frames, and the deformed figurines are images I will take to my grave. Domenico, Roberto, and Rocco shared a bedroom at that time. Bunk beds and furniture were crammed into one space to house three growing bodies and all their belongings. One night, Gian and I had fallen asleep on the couch. Rocco was also asleep on the couch in the basement (I guess this habit runs in the family). Domenico had left his bed for ours and fallen asleep there. This was his idea, and his routine. Startled to my feet by a noise coming from the boys' bedroom, I ran towards it. Nothing prepared me for what I was about to walk into, or onto. Broken glass, barefoot, a trail leading to Roberto's bed. There he lay quietly, awake, and miraculously uninjured. Roberto's need for order and tidiness, once benign, had metastasized. With the exception of the furniture, Roberto had moved every object in the room to one corner. Wall hangings had been pulled down and were piled one on top of the other. The electrical cord of the table lamp had been severed. Figurines without limbs lay piled like casualties after battle. Picture frames which had been displayed on the wardrobe cabinet had joined the carnage. Roberto had created a mountain of destruction, draped with bed linen and comforters, awaiting a proper burial.

As the house slept, Gian and I began the task of restoring order, Roberto-style. For the longest time, the bedroom remained barren with furniture only. We gradually reintroduced some wall hangings, a table lamp, and one framed picture on the night table. Rocco later moved into his own bedroom in the basement. I should have seen it coming. I should have known.

The unpredictable tendencies of people with autism continue to baffle the most brilliant of minds to this day. The behaviours of the community at large and people in particular are also unpredictable. Our own behaviours, at various stages in our lives, are yet to be lived and *understood*. But on some level it is also exciting not to know everything that is going to happen to us or how we will respond. Our lives, every morning, are handed to us like a blank sheet of paper or an unwrapped box of puzzle pieces. Yet I didn't always see the unpredictable nature of autism as a creative energy, as a force to foster personal and spiritual growth.

Like the parent who continues to weep over the living grave of the son she thought she gave birth to, I have moments of weakness. My fatigued mind is at times reduced to a narrow focus of the dark pieces of the autism puzzle - exclusion, discrimination, limitation. Parents of children who are developing normally have expectations that their children will achieve. Parents of children with autism hold the promise of a different success.

When supporting a person with autism, it is important for parents, guardians, caregivers and support workers to understand their own behaviour. I do not always reason why I do what I do, why I feel what I feel. Sometimes I am deeply disappointed and alarmed at my response to a situation. Roberto's graduation picture is another story I need to share.

Proud parents may frame their son's or daughter's graduation picture and hang it on the wall. They may give copies of this photograph to family and friends. When I received Roberto's graduation picture in the mail, I could not open it. For twelve months, I could not open it. My hesitation confused me. I was ashamed of myself. I have always been Roberto's cheerleader (and always will be). Why was I regressing into this pattern of negativity?

Roberto was not advancing to post-secondary education, employment, or a path of his own choosing. I knew that. I put the sealed envelope of his graduation picture on a shelf and left it there, hidden in plain sight. This was Roberto's last hooray, and I wanted it to last. Six months later, I purchased a frame. The pizza party inspired me to designate a day to open the envelope and frame his graduation picture. I chose my birthday.

The pizza party is a memory of Roberto's graduation that will fill your hearts with tenderness and your eyes with tears. You may want to get some tissue for this; I already have a handful ready. This story will touch you, deep within.

Roberto's graduation day was on Friday, May 26, 2015. The graduating class of 2015 was to receive their diplomas on Wednesday, June 24, 2015. Roberto was working through some challenging behaviours and medication changes at this time. I really wanted him to walk across the stage and receive his Certificate of Accomplishment. Roberto could not meet the requirements necessary to receive a Secondary School Diploma. His achievement, however, was just as impressive. I wanted him to have his moment to shine, just like Domenico had, two years prior.

Given the storm of 2013-2015, would Roberto be able to cope with all the changes that this graduation ceremony demanded? The ceremony was scheduled for 4:00 p.m. Five days a week Roberto looked forward to some quiet time before dinner after a busy day at school. So the timing of this ceremony would be change number one. He would miss dinner. This would be change number two. Roberto's bowel habits are virtually robotic. He usually has only one bowel movement a day, after dinner. If he attended the June 24 graduation ceremony, he would miss that movement. This would be change number three. He would be required to wear a gown (and a cap if he could tolerate it) for the duration of the ceremony over a minimum of two hours. This would be change number four. There would be no chance of taking pictures or socializing following the ceremony, if he got through it. We would fast forward the festivities to dinner, three hours later than usual. This would be change number five. Once home, there would be no time to reminisce about the high points of the ceremony. Roberto would need to make a beeline to the washroom and bathtub, immediately. This would be change number six. A half-day absence from his day program would be required to attend the ceremony. This would be change number seven. Roberto is extremely sensitive to change. It scares him. Could I impose all these changes, even with support, and expect him to be successful?

I had countless conversations with Roberto's teacher on how to best commemorate this milestone until it finally became crystal clear to us both. This was Roberto's achievement, his moment. His graduation ceremony had to be *meaningful to him*. I asked Roberto's teacher if we could simply have a quiet pizza party at the school. I asked her permission to invite some of Roberto's inner circle. Rocco, who had finished his first year of college, took the day off work to join us. Jennifer, who was in her final year of secondary school, missed the last part of her period three class. Gian was unable to leave the job. Domenico stayed at his day program (in adherence to his routine). I asked if they could present Roberto with a substitute Certificate of Accomplishment at the pizza party. I insisted on bringing the pizza. She insisted on bringing a vegetable tray (Roberto loves vegetables). We agreed on the date, the invited guests, the substitute certificate, the pizza, and the vegetable tray.

When Rocco and I walked into the classroom, I could not believe my eyes. If you are tissue-ready, pull up a cloud and read on. This moment in Roberto's life is heaven-sent.

The classroom was transformed into a party room - tablecloths, balloons, a spread of all Roberto's favourite food (meatballs, chicken fingers, beverages, delicatessen trays, fruit, and yes, vegetables). Excuse me for a minute (tissue break). A twenty-four inch cake, elevated on a pedestal, had these words: "Congratulations on your graduation, Roberto". A picture collage of Roberto with peers and teachers was framed and showcased. My pizza was in good company. The school chaplain approached me and explained how the graduation ceremony would proceed as Roberto emerged, wearing a blue graduation gown and cap (tissue break).

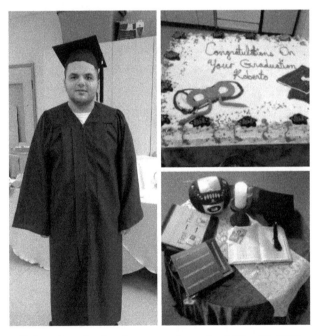

Roberto's graduation from secondary school, May 25, 2015

As a group (teachers, classmates, principal, guests), we gathered in the chapel. Chairs were arranged in a circle. At the centre of the room, they set up a small table with all items that personalize Roberto - CD player (loves calming music), PECS binder (his voice), school visual schedule (First → Then binder format), Bible, candle. The school chaplain started to talk. She asked all of us to raise our hands towards Roberto and then guided us in prayer (tissue break). She invited teachers and classmates to say out loud what they liked most about Roberto. The principal then presented Roberto with his Certificate of Accomplishment and offered him a sincere handshake. Once back in the classroom, we partied. Roberto smiled the entire time. He was present in the moment. He was celebrated and respected for who he is and for what he achieved and he knew it. He felt it, deep within. He was so happy.

How could I have predicted this outpouring of Christian love and generosity? The *respect* extended to Roberto will forever serve as a shining example of what we can do when we come together for a common purpose. *Compassion* and *understanding* of the behaviours of others and oneself leads to *respect*.

*Respect* is a piece of the autism puzzle that is not always found. People with autism deserve to be treated as valued members of society. *Understanding* the challenges they shoulder every single day and every single night, week after month after year, affords them favour and consideration. Reverence for all life should be upheld, for the love of God, for His name's sake.

One school bus company did not see it that way. It was Roberto's final year of secondary school. His transportation to and from school was a yellow, twenty-passenger school bus. The bus was equipped with harnesses and seat belts for younger riders who were scheduled to ride on later routes. But these seatbelts and harnesses brought Roberto's sensory system to a boiling point of visual overstimulation. Five weeks into the school year the morning bus driver said she had a problem with Roberto. He would stand up while the bus was in transit to unfasten the harnesses and seatbelts. As she approached Roberto in frustration, he was fast at work, unbuckling. She then turned to me and asked me to make him stop. I started to explain how OCD and SPD can manifest. She picked up her two-way radio and called the dispatcher of the bus company. As she was describing Roberto's non-compliance, I could hear the dispatcher's voice through the radio communication system. Instructions barked out, threatening to issue a pink slip if Roberto did not sit down and leave the belts alone. A pink slip is a written warning to riders that their bussing privileges will be suspended if appropriate behaviour is not exercised. Three pink slips and you walk. I asked if I could speak with the dispatcher. I wanted to give her a window into the autistic mind. Wendy's voice could be heard informing the driver that the radio communication system was for company employees only. While this one-sided dialogue ensued, Roberto had unbuckled all the harnesses and belts, sat down in his regular seat, and fastened his own seat belt. I assured the driver that I would call Wendy to problem-solve as she drove off with Roberto. In the time it took me to walk up my driveway, look up the telephone number of the bus company, and dial the number, Wendy was no longer available to talk with me. I was directed to take up my concerns with the School Board Transportation Department. I did so, immediately.

After several telephone menu selections and transfers to various departments, I finally spoke with Sharon in the Transportation Department. As I explained Roberto's challenging behaviour, Sharon, who had initially been defensive, actually listened. She first presented no options. Roberto had been assigned to the only route in our area and the only bus. In my dissatisfaction, I decided that I would drive Roberto to school for the remainder of the school year. I was not about to compromise his wellbeing or ability to successfully transition to day programming in eight months. Sharon found an alternative. A white, five-passenger minivan could pick Roberto up in the mornings. He would be the only rider and the drive would be direct. I was relieved, and grateful. It was Wednesday. This change was not possible until Monday. Sharon wanted me to talk to Roberto, asking him to manage for Thursday and Friday. I offered Sharon an analogy to help her understand why he could not cope. I asked her to imagine that she was to provide Roberto with vision correction lenses. She would not have his prescription glasses ready until Monday. In the short-term, she would give him another pair of glasses and expect him to be able to see through them. Asking him to ride in the yellow school bus until the white minivan was available was the same as asking him to see out of glasses that were not his.

The afternoon driver, also of a twenty-passenger school bus, also with harnesses and seat belts, extended *compassion* and *respect* to Roberto. He supported Roberto and his challenging behaviours. He took it upon himself to unfasten the harnesses and seat belts before Roberto entered the bus. It was his idea. Once Roberto was dropped off, this gentle and caring man returned all belts to their pre-Roberto state. It took all of five minutes, he told me, and he did not want my apology. It was not a big deal, he assured me. I should have asked Wendy to issue Roberto a blue slip instead of pink. Blue is the colour for autism.

Roberto's compromised sensory system graduated with him. Transportation to his day program was also by bus, also with seat-belts. He would stand while the bus was moving in order to fasten and then unfasten the seatbelts. The response to Roberto's behaviour did not travel down the same dead end street as the school transportation company. Clemency from the transportation manager carried hope back to my heart. Ongoing communication and collaboration prevail to this day. In one e-mail correspondence, she referred to Domenico and Roberto as "the gentlemen". She set in motion a mindset and a message. Yes, they are gentle and caring men. Yes, they are capable men. They just need a little help and a lot of love to find their way in life. They need us to keep working on the autism puzzle. If not for the compassion of our local transportation company, Domenico and Roberto would have no means of accessing community services; it would be as if they have no legs.

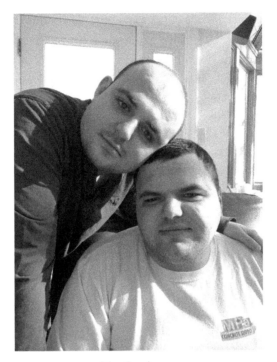

The Gentlemen

It has taken me twenty years to gather all the pieces of my broken heart and put them back together again. But now, I am whole. Thank you for spending this time with me. Let's recap.

*Acceptance*, the frame of the autism puzzle, lays the foundation upon which we can build a better world. *Faith* strengthens and sustains the frame. *Compassion, understanding,* and *respect* come together to form the centre of the puzzle, the core of the image. They outnumber and overpower all the dark pieces of the autism puzzle - intolerance, ignorance, discrimination, and greed. Say yes to diversity, say yes to inclusion, say yes to God. He is always listening.

With every hardship and every blessing, I put the pieces of autism and faith together. I built a life with God. The puzzle that I imagined God gave me in the doctor's office, two decades ago, was complete. Its image, like a kaleidoscope of hope and promise, became crystal clear. I can see it now in all its vitality and might. I bet you can already guess what the puzzle's image is (my readers are so smart)! It is the solution to the autism puzzle. It is what I have been looking for my entire life. It is a staircase to God.

Lesson learned - Drop your defences. Lift up your heart to God. Fold your hands in prayer and allow God to work through you. Put your trust in Him. God does not thrust us into troubled times to punish us no more than He carries us into times of plenty to reward us. God is transforming us, with every tear and every smile. Piece by piece, one step at a time, our understanding of ourselves and God will come together, in full view, and make us whole again.

# Chapter Twenty

## EVERY DAY IS A NEW DAY:
## CLOSE ENCOUNTERS OF THE BEST KIND

*Use me God. Show me how to take who I
am, who I want to be, and what I can do and
use it for a purpose greater than myself.*

**MARTIN LUTHER KING JR.**

I do not want a polished life of ease and privilege. No, thank you. I
do not think I will find God there. I want a roll-up-your-sleeves life
of substance and service. So, have I got what I wanted, or have I been
given what I needed?

I have played out this scenario in the sanctity of my private thoughts
a thousand times over. I imagine God coming to town with an entou-
rage of rock star status. He will grant each person their will, not His.
Ask, and God, the ultimate provider, will deliver. As line-ups begin
to swell, I secure my place, determined to wait patiently for my turn,
however long. After what feels like an eternity, I am next. There I am,
virtually speechless. This is God, after all, who sits across the table
from me. In reverence to Our Father through whom everything is
possible, I find the courage to speak. You are probably wondering if
I would ask God to take autism away. I guess this is tempting, but

no, not a chance. I would ask for nothing, because God has given me everything. *Your will, God, is my will.* I would offer Him my gratitude for the life-altering gifts of autism. Well, I would try.

Lesson learned - Let God be God!

I have always described autism as both basic and complex. As Domenico's and Roberto's primary caregiver, I have assumed the responsibility for their basic needs such as dressing, bathing, nutrition, active living, quality leisure time, and personal hygiene as well as dental, vision, and medical care. I must say I am becoming very comfortable with the razor's edge. Roberto rocks the chin strap and cleans up quite nicely, thank you very much.

Conventional wisdom would have it that I will teach them more than they could ever teach me, but in reality, the opposite is true. Through Domenico and Roberto, I have learned two fundamental life lessons. First, for the human heart to be complete and grow strong, the human heart must carry both celebration and sorrow. These polarized emotions are so intimately connected when living with autism that every single day I find myself laughing and crying at the same time. The second life lesson is perhaps even greater than the first. I have learned that when we bring together our diverse abilities for a common purpose, we can build a bridge to God. Together, we can grow in faith. Facing an uncertain future with a certain God, I am no longer afraid but rather have found peace and opportunity in the darkest of places: in the autistic mind.

Yes, the basic milestones that come inherently to most will never be celebrated by my sons - a sobering thought, I know. In fact, they will never have the presence of mind to make real choices. Having the cognitive ability to make choices for one's life is indeed a gift. Domenico and Roberto will never marry, but they walk hand in hand with God. They will never develop employable skills, yet they are doing God's work. My sons will never operate a motor vehicle, but they can help drive others to their full potential. No child will call them Dad, but they are Fathers of Peace, strong and true.

I have chosen to trust God, believing that God's purpose is greater than my pain. Autism has given me a window into the gifts of living with what may appear as insurmountable challenges and the view literally brings me to my knees, second to none. Perhaps you can relate. Perhaps the mountains you climb every day were put there, not to challenge you, but rather to give you a better view of your life and your purpose, to help you achieve clarity of thought.

It seems that I have been in constant pursuit of the meaning of my life for the past forever. I wanted to be a nurse and worked hard to get accepted into the program of my choice, so why did I quit? This question has tormented me for most of my adult life. Perhaps I turned away from my dream in order to walk into the will of God. Perhaps what I wanted from life and what God needed from my life differed. I know I have never worked so hard, for so long, for something that hurts so much, so why have I not given up on autism? Is it possible that God is the answer? Without even registering for the course, I remain a student in God's classroom. My greatest assignment was given on January 19, 1996, the day I received Domenico's diagnosis.

Over my lifetime and especially during the past twenty-five years, God has sent His people to instruct me, to inspire me, to challenge me, to comfort me, to protect me, and to just be my friend. I am grateful for the work God has brought to my hands to teach me that I am able. I am blessed to hear His voice in the absence of the spoken word to remind me that I will be okay. Empowered by the sanctity of His plan and eternally humbled to be in His service, I choose God. Through His select few, I feel God's presence. Through my sons Domenico and Roberto, I see God's perfect image.

*When I go for a walk with Roberto, hand in hand, I know it is You, Father, holding onto me. When Domenico's eyes awaken from sound slumber to sweet smiles, I know it is You, Father, smiling at me.*

What was once my deepest sorrow is now my greatest joy. As challenging as a life with autism is, I would not trade it for any rose-coloured world. I do not think I would learn as much. The non-verbal world has translated into a realization of my true potential and purpose that can never be silenced. *This is for you, God; I labour for You.*

I am just an ordinary person living an extraordinary life because God is there, God is everywhere. On the wings of autism, in all its glory, I soar to purpose high!

# Epilogue

## P.S. YOU ARE MY FAVOURITE SUBJECTS

---

*What I do, you cannot do, but what you do,*
*I cannot do. The needs are great, and none of*
*us, including me, can ever do great things. But*
*we can all do small things, with great love, and*
*together we can do something wonderful.*

---

**MOTHER TERESA**

Dear Gian, Domenico, Roberto, Rocco, and Jennifer,

My favourite subjects in secondary school were Mathematics, Science, and English. I worked hard. I earned the grades. I still maintain a high regard for formal education. Always will. What I learned in Mathematics, however, did not teach me to count my blessings. Science did not provide the formula for a fulfilling life. I never read the *Book of Life* in English class because it does not exist. The most valued lessons, the greatest skills I learned to this day, I learned from you. You are my favourite subjects.

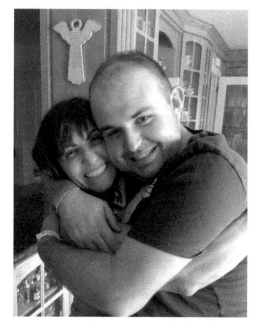

Morning squeeze with Domenico, The Stud Muffin

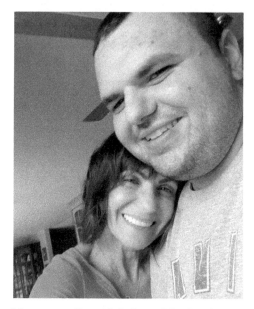

Afternoon smiles with Roberto, The Gentle Giant

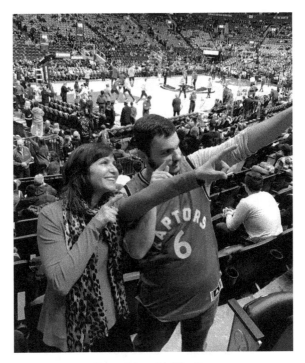

Date night with The Roc

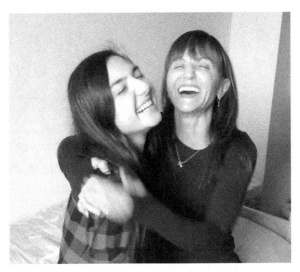

University residence, First year, first visit with Jennifer

I wanted to be a nurse. I wanted to minister to the needs of others. During times of infirmity, I wanted to be there to comfort, to counsel, to be a friend. You gave me those moments. You are my quiet river. You are my anchor. You are the antidote for my ailing self-esteem. You are my chosen career.

I made a promise to myself: a promise to demonstrate my love. If opportunities did not present themselves, I promised to create them.

That is the reason I wrote this book. I did it for God. I did it for you. God brought the six of us together for a reason. God's plans never fail.

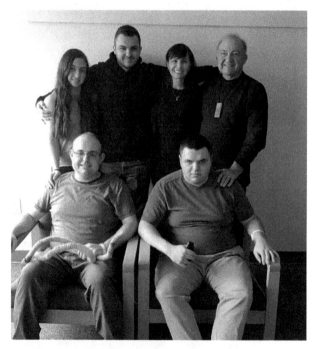

They take my breath away, Family is everything, 2017

We are but flesh and blood. We refuse, however, to exist as a mere shell of a human being. We refuse to schlep through life like walking corpses. No way! We choose the road less travelled, the narrow gate.

Life is not supposed to be easy. Life is supposed to matter. We choose to make it matter.

Nobody, including us, knows where we will be tomorrow. But we are together, right here, right now, in this moment, and there is no other place I would rather be than right here with you.

We fear and we are fearless. We weaken and we are fierce. We tire and we rebuild. We laugh, we cry, we work, we rest. We are family.

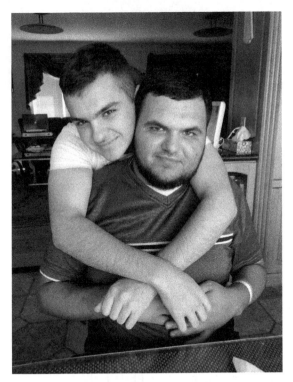

Rocco and Roberto, Heart to heart

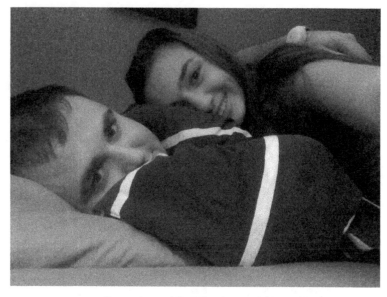

Domenico and Jennifer, A united force

Life will give and life will take. Gian, I asked God to never separate us. I want to be with you until the day after forever. God said there is a "Season and a time for every purpose under heaven. Trust me." *I do, Father.* Domenico and Roberto, I begged God to let me bury you. Who will care for you when I die? God said, "It does not work like that; leave that to me." *I will, Father.* Rocco and Jennifer, I asked God to bless you as graciously as you have blessed me. "You are welcome my child," God rejoiced.

Gian, Domenico, Roberto, Rocco, and Jennifer, God said, "Leave the hard stuff to me." We should listen. I know that with God we are in good hands. I know that with you, I have it all.

Always and forever, I love you. Amen!

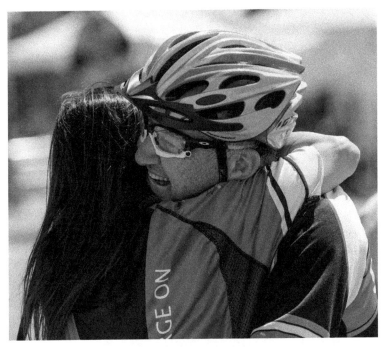

Never let you go, Finish line, 2016

Last Lesson - For me, the two most enabling human attributes are adaptability and perseverance. The two most empowering human emotions are love and hope. The two most destructive human dispositions are hate and fear.

Life will continue to humble us. Life will continue to challenge us. Do not be afraid. Life is beautiful. Not because it is perfect. Not because it is without struggle. Life is beautiful because it affords us the opportunity to grow through adversity and find God. I am praying for you. I am praying that you commit to change and endurance. I am praying that you follow your dreams with all your heart, mind and spirit. Please never raise your arms in defeat. Please never point your finger in defence. And above all, whatever you do, wherever you go, always remember to look up. God bless you, my friends.

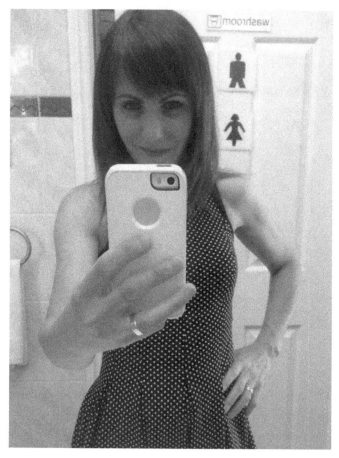

Me again, Still small, 2016

# FINAL THOUGHTS

## What They Would Say With Words
## Domenico and Roberto Sansalone

*Maybe I can't change the world, but I can
affect the people around me; and if they in turn
do the same and affect those around them,
then, together we can change the world.*

**AARON SHEPPARD**

Call me old-fashioned. Call me foolish. I would go as far as to say I am a little naïve. But I still believe that love will get me through the hardest of times. Domenico and Roberto, they are love. And they say it best. I want them to have the last word. *Gentlemen, I know you are afraid but they are good people. It's your turn to talk.*

> Dear everyone, our message to you is one of promise and praise. It comes from a sacred place, our hearts.

> We may not understand everything, but we understand love. Where science and medicine and politics and education end, love endures and empowers. Love never ends.

Thank you for the love. Thank you for including us in your conversations and welcoming us into your social circles. Thank you for speaking to us both in your language (with words) so we learn, and in our language (with pictures) so we understand. For all the times you smile at us and others with disabilities, we notice. Your smiles tell us it is okay to be our messy, beautiful selves, free from reproach or reprisal. For all the times you are our voice, fearless and determined, we hear you. You speak to educate and enlighten. Many listen. Positive change comes from your advocacy. For all you do without speaking a word, we see you. You build bridges and open doors. Your working hands and caring ways make a difference.

So let's keep going. Let's dare to build a better world. If you are meeting us for the first time, look for the light in our eyes and the potential in our hands. When you hear our sounds, listen for the will of our spirits and the song in our hearts. As we labour together, recognize that we are the same as much as we are different. Rise up to the virtues of humility and charity. And most of all be loving and kind, as often as you can and to as many people as you can. Know that you will always delight in your decision to do the right thing and, truth be told, it could have been you.

P.S. Autism speaks!

CPSIA information can be obtained
at www.ICGtesting.com
Printed in the USA
LVHW01s0440211117
557143LV00001B/37/P